Overcome Diabetes

How to Reverse Type 2 Diabetes without Drugs:

4-Step Quick Start Guide

By James Strand

© 2017 reversediabetes101.com

All Rights Reserved

Publisher's Note: The information contained herein is not intended to replace the services of a trained health professional or to be a substitute for individual medical advice. You should consult with your health care professional in regards to any matter relating to your health, and in particular, any matter that may require diagnosis or medical attention.

Uncontrolled high or low blood sugar levels are dangerous, and you need to seek immediate medical care for these conditions. If you are being treated for diabetes, any changes in your existing medications are not advised without first consulting a medical professional. Additionally, any changes in your diet and exercise practices should follow the guidelines of a medical professional who has personally examined you.

Material Connection Disclosure: The publisher of this book may have an affiliate relationship and or another material connection to the providers of goods and services mentioned in this book. If you purchase any of these items contained herein, the publisher may receive additional compensation.

First Edition 2017 (015p)

Overcome Diabetes--How to Reverse Type 2 Diabetes without Drugs:
4-Step Quick Start Guide

By James Strand
Copyright © 2017 reversediabetes101.com
All Rights Reserved

Published by:
reversediabetes101.com
1201 Military Dr. Ste. 2
PMB #279
Benton, AR 72015

ISBN: 978-1542547345

www.reversediabetes.com

Table of Contents

Step 1: Understand the Problem of Diabetes

Hard Facts about Diabetes

Diabetes is a major health crisis. Over 420 million people around the world are suffering from diabetes. The total number of those with diabetes has quadrupled in the last 35 years. At this time, a little more than one in every 12 people has the disease. Diabetes is spreading worldwide. Diabetes was once a disease of the West, but it is now in every country. Experts predict by the year 2035 the number of people in the world with diabetes will approach 600 million.

The Unrelenting March of Diabetes

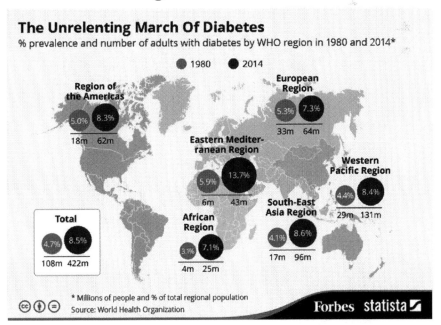

"The Unrelenting Global March of Diabetes" Licensed by CC BY-ND 2.0
Infographic http://www.forbes.com/sites/niallmccarthy/2016/04/07/the-unrelenting-global-march-of-diabetes-infographic/

There are also millions of people with a condition known as prediabetes. According to the US Centers for Disease Control and Prevention, there are an estimated 89 million people in the U.S. have prediabetes–and almost 90% of them do not know it. In a few years, 15%-30% percent of people who have prediabetes will have it turn into type 2 diabetes. It is very likely that you or someone you know will have their life dramatically impacted by diabetes.

Those who have prediabetes can almost always prevent it from turning into type 2 diabetes. A large percentage of those who already have type 2 diabetes can have their diabetes go into remission or reversal. This book will provide information about how thousands of people have changed their lives and prevented type 2 diabetes, or they had it reversed and go in remission so they no longer needed drugs to control it.

The Rise of Diabetes and Obesity Are Linked

More than half of Americans are overweight. This includes at least one in five children who are above the normal weight for their age. Obesity is a term applied to overweight people with an excessive amount of body fat. One in four Americans is obese. There can be some medical reasons for obesity, but nutritionists and health experts say the main reason for the increase in obesity is a poor diet and physical inactivity.

Excess body weight is a result of an imbalance of calories consumed versus calories burned through physical activity. If you consume more calories than you expend through exercise and daily activities, you gain weight. Your body stores calories that you do not need for energy as fat.

The rise in obesity goes hand in hand with the rise in diabetes. It is not true to say all overweight people will develop diabetes. Many overweight people never develop diabetes. Weight is not always a factor present in every case of diabetes. However, many overweight individuals develop diabetes. Being overweight does seem to be an important factor in most cases of diabetes.

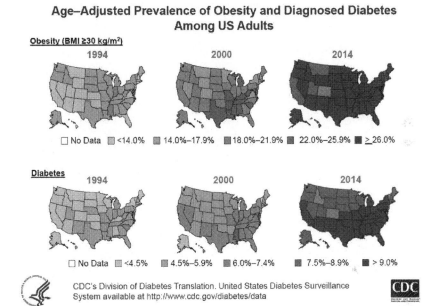

Age–Adjusted Prevalence of Obesity and Diagnosed Diabetes Among US Adults

Obesity (BMI ≥30 kg/m²)

1994   2000   2014

☐ No Data   ▨ <14.0%   ▧ 14.0%–17.9%   ▩ 18.0%–21.9%   ■ 22.0%–25.9%   ■ ≥26.0%

Diabetes

1994   2000   2014

☐ No Data   ▨ <4.5%   ▩ 4.5%–5.9%   ■ 6.0%–7.4%   ■ 7.5%–8.9%   ■ > 9.0%

CDC's Division of Diabetes Translation. United States Diabetes Surveillance System available at http://www.cdc.gov/diabetes/data

CDC

Information in the previous infographic was provided by the United States (US) Centers for Disease Control and Prevention (CDC). The maps illustrate over the last 20 years the increase in obesity among US adults and the increase of diabetes goes together hand-in-hand.

The first group of three maps shows the prevalence of obesity for the years 1994, 2000 and 2014. In 1994, the majority of states show that less than 14% of adults were obese. In the year 2014, the percentage rose to between 22% and 26%.

The second group of three maps shows the prevalence of diabetes for the years 1994, 2000 and 2014. In 1994, approximately half of all states showed about 4.5% of adults had diabetes. In the year 2014, the percentages rose to between 7.5% and 9%.

These numbers are high, but they only tell part of the story. If undiagnosed diabetes numbers were included, the number of people in the US affected by diabetes the numbers would be higher.

From the statistics available from the CDC and other organizations, it is rather easy to conclude the dramatic increase in diabetes is directly linked to the rise in obesity.

The number of new cases of diabetes has grown dramatically over the past few years, and it appears that the increase in new cases will continue to grow during the next few years as well. In the U.S., the greatest number of new cases of diabetes affects people after they reach the age of 45. However, younger age groups including children are also seeing an increase in diabetes. The numbers in the chart below represent new cases of diabetes for one year.

New Cases of Diagnosed Diabetes in the U.S. Aged 20 Years or Older

Number of New Diabetes Cases By Age	Number of New Diabetes Cases	Rate of New Diabetes Cases per 1,000
20-44	371,000	3.6
45-64	892,000	12
65 or older	400,000	11.5
Total	1.7 million	7.8

Source: 2010-2012 National Health Interview Survey, 2009-2012 National Health and Nutrition Examination Survey, and 2012 U.S. Census data.

Several other factors may contribute to diabetes such as age and genetics. However, inactivity and poor eating practices appear to be the main culprits in weight gain and the rising levels of diabetes in the U.S. and around the world. If these lifestyle conditions are changed, we could see the total number of new cases of diabetes start to decrease. When this happens, the health of millions of individuals around the world will improve. It is clear more action is required, sooner than later, to address these dual health care crises of obesity and diabetes.

What Is Diabetes?

Diabetes Mellitus. The clinical name for the disease of diabetes is a combination of the Greek word diabetes, which means to pass through, and the Latin word mellitus, which means honey or sweet. This came about from the observation that the urine of diabetics was sweet and attracted ants.

Diabetes is a metabolic disease that causes the blood sugar or glucose levels in the body's bloodstream to become excessively high.

After eating food containing sugars and starches, these carbohydrates are quickly broken down into the simple sugar glucose by the digestive system. The pancreas is a large gland behind the stomach. As glucose passes from the digestive system to the bloodstream, the pancreas releases insulin to lower the blood sugar levels. The insulin secreted by pancreas causes the cells in the body to use the glucose to produce energy. The energy from glucose provides the energy the body needs to perform daily activities.

Insulin acts like a key within the cells that allows the cells to break down the glucose and use the energy. Insulin causes the blood sugar levels to return to normal within two hours of eating.

Someone with diabetes still has high levels of blood sugar after two hours from eating. In a normal person, when glucose is not used up as energy, it often gets stored as fat. Diabetes causes some of this excess sugar to be reabsorbed from the blood and excreted in the urine.

One of the early signs of prediabetes and diabetes is weight loss, hunger and fatigue. Because the body does not get enough energy from glucose, it gets energy by breaking down fat, muscles and other tissues in the body. Even though a person eats more and more sugary foods, he still feels hungry because the cells cannot use the food for energy.

If left untreated, high blood sugar levels in the blood will have a damaging effect on the cells of the body. The complications of uncontrolled diabetes include blindness, kidney disease, amputations and premature death.

Diabetes is the seventh leading cause of death. Diabetes is also a factor in the deaths of many people who die from strokes and heart disease. Diabetes is a serious condition that needs medical attention. If ignored, the consequences of uncontrolled diabetes will be dire.

There are three major types diabetes: type 1 diabetes, type 2 diabetes and gestational diabetes. In type 1 diabetes, the body cannot make insulin. In type 2 diabetes, the body makes insulin, but it is not working properly. Gestational diabetes sometimes temporarily appears during pregnancy.

Approximately 90% of diabetes is type 2 diabetes and 5% is type 1 diabetes. The other 5% of diabetes cases are composed of gestational diabetes and other rarer types of diabetes not mentioned here.

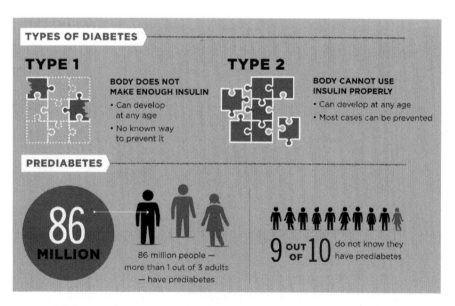

US Centers for Disease Control and Prevention (CDC). Infographic: https://www.cdc.gov/diabetes/library/socialmedia/infographics.html

Type 1 Diabetes

Type 1 diabetes was previously called juvenile diabetes, but this term is no longer widely used. Type 1 diabetes can affect people of all ages, but most new cases are found in people before the age of 20.

Type 1 diabetes results from problems with the pancreas. The pancreas malfunctions and can no longer make the proper amount of insulin. Without the right amount of insulin, sugar in the blood is not used by the cells. This causes the sugar levels to build up in the blood.

Type 1 diabetes is a dangerous condition that requires the injection of insulin to sustain life. Once the insulin is injected, the body's cells use insulin to produce energy properly. This returns blood sugar levels to normal. However, the person with Type 1 diabetes must continue to take insulin.

Type 1 diabetes is not reversible, but there is hope that in the near future a cure will be available. There is experimental pancreas transplantation research underway that looks promising.

Type 2 Diabetes

90% of all diabetes is type 2 diabetes. Type 2 diabetes was previously called adult onset diabetes, but this term is no longer popular. Over the past few years, there is an alarming rise in the number of children who develop type 2 diabetes. However, the largest number of new cases of diabetes occurs in people over the age of 45.

Type 1 and type 2 diabetes are very different. In Type 1 diabetes, the pancreas makes no insulin. In type 2 diabetes, the pancreas makes insulin. Often in type 2 diabetes, the pancreas produces more insulin than in a normal person. In type 2 diabetes, it is not the lack of insulin that causes the problem. It is the inability of the body's cells to use insulin. This condition is called insulin resistance.

Insulin resistance keeps the cells from using glucose in the blood. This excess glucose stays in the blood and is eventually reabsorbed by the kidneys. Then, it passes out of the body in the urine. However, the overall level of sugar in the blood remains higher than normal

Doctors usually prescribe oral medications to control the blood sugar levels in type 2 diabetes. The medicines treat the symptom of high blood sugar. This is important and can remove the excess sugar in the blood. This slows down or stops additional complications of the disease. However, the treatment of the symptoms of diabetes does nothing to reverse the underlying problems causing the disease.

As type 2 diabetes advances, the pancreas may begin to malfunction and stop producing insulin. This progression of the disease may take several years, or it may occur sooner. When this happens, insulin injections are required to control high blood sugar the same as in type 1 diabetes.

Early intervention after the initial onset of type 2 diabetes will prevent complications. If you make changes in your diet and exercise habits at this point, it is likely you can see the full remission or reversal of the disease.

If you are serious about reversing your type 2 diabetes, it is important to develop an action plan. Once you have a proven action plan, you need to start following it as quickly as possible. By reducing the number of calories eaten, losing weight and exercising more often, most cases of type 2 diabetes can be reversed.

Studies have shown that when Type 2 diabetics lose weight, eat better and increase their physical activity, they can reduce their insulin resistance and other underlying causes of diabetes.

Taking action sooner than later may make it possible for you to see tremendous results in only a few weeks or a few months. Even if you cannot reverse your diabetes completely, you can gain better control of your blood sugar levels.

Gestational Diabetes

Gestational diabetes mellitus (GDM) is a temporary condition that occurs when there are higher blood glucose levels than normal in a woman's body during pregnancy. Gestational diabetes usually goes away on its own once the woman has given birth. Gestational diabetes may occur in 4% to 9% of pregnancies. Women with gestational diabetes are at a higher risk of complications during pregnancy and delivery. Testing for gestational diabetes is a routine procedure during pregnancy.

Prediabetes

Prediabetes is a condition with higher than normal blood sugar levels, but these levels are not high enough to classify as type 2 diabetes. People who have prediabetes have a greater risk of developing type 2 diabetes in a few years. The good news is prediabetes can be reversed and prevented from turning into type 2 diabetes with the proper lifestyle changes. It is a true saying, "an ounce of prevention with is worth a pound of cure."

What Causes Diabetes?

The specific cause of diabetes remains somewhat elusive to researchers. However, many factors are considered important in the onset of the disease. The factors that cause type 1 diabetes are different from type 2 diabetes factors.

It might surprise some to find out that eating sugar is not one of the causes of diabetes. Sugar consumption may cause obesity, but it is not a direct factor in the cause of diabetes. Excessive sugar consumption is not good for a person with diabetes because they already have too much sugar in their blood, but it is not the cause of diabetes.

Medical science is trying to figure out why some are affected by diabetes while others remain unaffected. The causes of different types of diabetes may be different, but they all result in high blood sugar.

Factors in the Onset of Type 1 Diabetes

It is thought that Type 1 diabetes is an autoimmune disease, which means that the immune system of the body acts against the cells of the pancreas, thus hampering the production of insulin. A susceptibility to developing this type of diabetes may occur in families. Certain kinds of viral infections may also cause it.

Factors in the Onset of Type 2 Diabetes

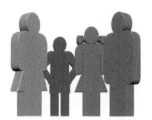

Hereditary Factor: A strong genetic link is suspected in type 2 diabetes, which means that it has a tendency of running in families. Those who have a history of diabetes in their family background are 25 percent more susceptible to developing diabetes.

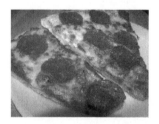

Dietary Factor: Modern eating habits comprise largely of consuming foods containing high-calorie carbohydrates and fats such as pizza, cheeseburgers, fries, drinks, ice cream, cookies, snacks and so on. Bad food choices have helped increase diabetes rates around the world.

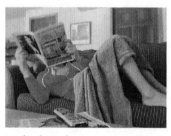

Sedentary Lifestyle: The modern lifestyle that many people lead today involves less physical work and long hours of sitting during work. After work, leisure activities are often just as sedentary. Lying on the couch watching TV or knocking back beers at the bar does not count as a core exercise or bicep training. If you live an inactive and sedentary lifestyle, research has revealed that you have a much higher chance of developing type 2 diabetes and its related problems.

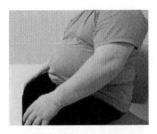

Excessive Weight: Excessive weight is the most important risk factor for type 2 diabetes. Fat cells play a role in insulin resistance that hampers the metabolism of glucose. This leads to hyperglycemia (an excess of glucose in the blood) which ultimately results in diabetes.

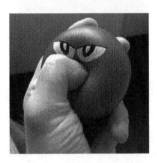

Stress Factor: Most people encounter a high amount of stress in their jobs or in their day-to-day activities. The body's metabolism is adversely affected by a chaotic and irregular lifestyle. Even emotional stress such as worry, anxiety and grief may cause changes in the blood sugar levels, leading to the disease.

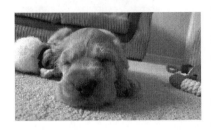

Lack of Adequate Sleep. There is growing evidence that not sleeping well can contribute to the development of diabetes. Lack of sleep increases the stress hormone cortisol, increases appetite and elevates blood sugar.

Getting the right amount of sleep can improve blood sugar control. Studies show that sleeping about eight hours a night is best for most people.

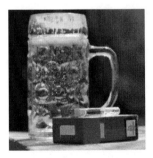

Additional Factors: Excessive alcoholic beverage consumption can cause weight gain that increases the risk of diabetes. Smoking is also an additional factor. These factors can be completely eliminated by not smoking or consuming alcoholic beverages. If you drink excessively, or if your smoke, you can choose not to. Other factors such as high blood pressure and age can contribute to the onset of type 2 diabetes.

Are You at Risk for Diabetes?

What is Your Body Mass Index (BMI)

> *Adolphe Quetelet, a Belgian mathematician who was born in 1796, invented the calculation for BMI. He proposed that people's weight could be classified relative to an ideal weight for their height. To this day, the Body Mass Index is also referred to as the Quetelet index.*

If you are overweight, you have a higher risk of developing diabetes. This is why it is important to keep an eye on your weight and your Body Mass Index (BMI). BMIs between 18.5 and 25 are healthy.

The Body Mass Index (BMI)	
Below 18.5	Underweight
18.5 to 24.9	Healthy weight
25 to 29.9	Overweight
30 to 39.9	Obese
40 to 49.9	Morbidly Obese
50+	Super Obese

There are a number of online BMI calculators you can use to calculate your BMI. Here is one from the National Heart, Lung and Blood Institute. It is simple to use. Enter your height and weight and it will use the * BMI formula to calculate your BMI.

http://www.nhlbi.nih.gov/health/educational/lose_wt/BMI/bmicalc.htm

*The formula for calculating BMI: BMI = weight-kg/(height-m)^2. Where kg is weight in kilograms, m is height in meters, 2 means squared (m x m).

BMI can be used to get an approximate value for body fat. This formula is adjusted for age and gender. Most people gain body fat as they age. Women have slightly more body fat than men.

Body Fat Percentage = 1.2 × BMI + 0.23 × age − 5.4 − 10.8 × gender
(where gender is 0 if female and 1 if male)

There are also some alternative ways to measure your body fat. Your health care provider may have a handheld BMI machine that gives an instant reading. Another method is to use a caliper device that pinches the skin and gives a skinfold measurement. Various skinfold measurements are taken, and the BMI is calculated from them.

Most People in the US Are Overweight or Obese

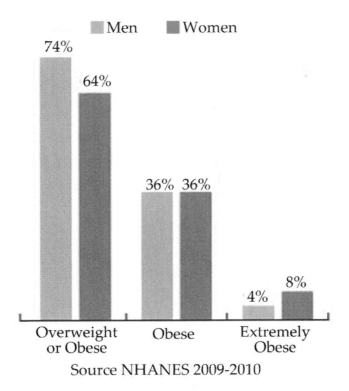

Estimated Percentage Of
Overweight People by Sex

Source NHANES 2009-2010

US Government statistics from the National Health and Nutrition Examination Survey (NHANES) has shown that 74% of men and 64% of women in the US are either overweight or obese. In this chart, a BMI of 25-29.9 is categorized as Overweight. A BMI between 30 and 39.9 is Obese. A BMI greater than 40 is Extremely Obese.

Waist Size and Type 2 Diabetes Risk

Although waist circumference and Body Mass Index (BMI) are interrelated, waist circumference provides another independent prediction of the high risk of developing type 2 diabetes. Waist circumference measurement is particularly useful in people who are categorized as normal or overweight on the BMI scale.

Waist Circumference Diabetes Type 2
High Risk Assessments

Men: Waist size > 40 inches (102 cm)   ***Asian Men:** Waist size >35 inches (89 cm)

Women: Waist size > 35 inches (89 cm)   **Asian Women:** Waist size Waist size > 31 inches (79 cm)

*Researchers recommend smaller waist circumferences be used for Asian populations to determine diabetes risks. The symbol ">" is a mathematical shortcut symbol that means greater than.

Truncal Obesity is a term given to the common term "belly fat." The term refers to the fat stored in the abdominal area rather than on the arms, legs or other places. Abdominal fat can be fat just under the skin or a deeper internal fat called visceral fat. Visceral fat makes up the majority of abdominal fat. Visceral fat is fat packed around the liver, pancreas and kidneys and other organs inside the abdominal cavity.

The common "pot belly" is composed mostly of visceral fat. Your waist circumference is a good indicator of how much visceral fat you have. As your waist gets bigger, your risk for type 2 diabetes increases.

Abdominal obesity and visceral fat are associated with increased risks of high cholesterol, poor physical conditioning, increased risk of diabetes and heart disease. Abdominal obesity is more prevalent in men than women.

Are There Any Early Signs of Diabetes or Prediabetes?

A few symptoms of diabetes are manifested in the early stage (or prediabetes phase). About one-third of people who have diabetes remain unaware of their high blood sugar levels. When the early signs of diabetes are present, they are often confused with symptoms of other health problems. Let us look into some of the warning signs of diabetes.

Frequent Urination and Thirst

A common symptom exhibited in the early stages of Type 1 and type 2 diabetes is frequent urination (polyuria) and dehydration (polydipsia). When the glucose in the blood increases above normal, the reabsorption of sugar from the blood by the kidneys is incomplete. This excess sugar hinders water absorption by the kidneys. This extra water results in frequent urination. The increase in the frequency of urination causes excessive fluid loss. Ultimately, dehydration occurs, causing increased thirst.

Increased Appetite

Another warning sign of Type 1 or type 2 diabetes is increased appetite. Normally, glucose is used for energy by the body for its various functions. In type 2 diabetes, it is not used properly by the cells and remains in the blood. When the cells sense they no longer have energy and cannot get it from glucose, it sends messages to the brain to eat something to get more energy. This is why diabetes causes hunger (polyphagia).

Unusual Weight Loss

A person who has diabetes or prediabetes often suffers from unusual weight loss, even without trying. This is caused by excessive loss of sugar (glucose) in the urine. When the body cannot use sugar for energy, it starts using fats and proteins as its source of energy.

Feelings of Fatigue

Diabetes and prediabetes will cause a person to have excess sugar in their blood and not in their cells. As their body's cells are deprived from the energy in glucose, they will often experience feelings of increased fatigue. Physical ability is lowered and the person gets tired easily.

Numbness or Tingling in the Hands and Feet

Unchecked high sugar brings about damage to the nerves (neuropathy). This causes symptoms such as numbness or a tingling sensation in the hands and feet.

Vision Problems

Vision problems are more likely in people with diabetes and prediabetes. The increase in the blood sugar levels leads to changes in the shape of the eye lenses. If diabetes is uncontrolled for a long time, this can result in poor focusing power and blurred vision. Diabetes complications are the leading cause of blindness in the US.

Frequent Infections

The immune system of a person with diabetes or prediabetes is often lower than the immune system of a healthy person. This may be due to the presence of elevated glucose in the blood, which in turn hampers the proper functioning of white blood cells (leukocytes). This compromised immune system often results in frequent colds, flu and other infections like pneumonia. There may also be skin infections and yeast infections. In addition, cuts and wounds take longer to heal.

Tests for Diabetes and Prediabetes

In the US most types of blood sugar tests other than the HbA1c are measured in milligrams per deciliter (mg/dl). A milligram is very small (.000018) or 18/millionths of a teaspoon. A deciliter is about 3 1/3 ounces.

If you suspect you have diabetes or prediabetes, your doctor can perform tests to diagnose your situation. Uncontrolled blood sugar levels are dangerous and you need to get them under control as soon as possible. If you think you might have diabetes, do not try to diagnose and treat yourself. You need the help of a medical professional to walk you through the treatment options. This will ensure that you will avoid further complications of the disease.

Type of Test	Normal	Pre-Diabetes	Type 1 or Type 2 Diabetes
HbA1c Test (glycosylated hemoglobin)	4%-5.9%	5.6%-6.4%	6.5% or higher
Fasting Blood Sugar Test	80-99 mg/dl	100-125 mg/dl	126 mg/dl or higher
Oral Glucose Tolerance Test	139 mg/dl or lower	140-199 mg/dl	200 mg/dl or higher
Random Glucose Test (glucometer)	80-100 mg/dl	100-199 mg/dl	200 mg/dl or higher (plus symptoms)

In Canada, the UK and other countries blood sugar levels are measured in millimoles per liter (mmol/l). You can convert US blood sugars to the UK measurement by dividing the US number by 18. If a US blood sugar level of 90 is reported, then divide this by 18 and you will get the UK measurement of 5. The US number of 198 converts to 11 in UK units. If you see UK units, you can convert it back to US units by doing the opposite and multiplying it by 18.

HbA1c Test

HbA1c test often just called the A1c Test. The technical name is called a glycosylated hemoglobin test. This lab test requires that a sample of blood be drawn from a vein in the arm. It measures the amount of glucose sugar attached to the hemoglobin protein in red blood cells. The test shows the doctor the levels of glucose in the over the period of the last two or three months. From this number it can be determined how well, or not so well, blood sugar was controlled over time. The normal range for this test is measured in percentages. 4%-6% is normal. 6.5% or higher indicates diabetes. HbA1c is the preferred test most health care practitioners use to diagnose and manage diabetes over time.

Fasting Plasma Glucose Test (FPG)

The Fasting Plasma Glucose Test is also known as a Fasting Blood Sugar Test. This is a lab test that is performed on a sample of blood that is drawn from a vein in the arm. This test determines the amount of glucose in the plasma or liquid portion of the blood. This test is usually done the first thing in the morning after not eating or drinking anything for at least 8 hours. Readings over 126 mg/dl indicate diabetes. Readings between 100 and 125 mg/dl indicate prediabetes.

Oral Glucose Tolerance Test (OGTT)

The Oral Glucose Tolerance Test is a lab test taken from a sample of blood drawn from the arm. It checks to see if you can drink a special sugary drink and have your blood sugar return to normal within two hours. A sample of blood is taken before the test and another sample is taken at the end of the two hours. Readings over 200 mg/dl indicate diabetes. Readings between 140 and 199 mg/dl indicate prediabetes.

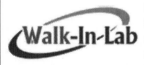 Diabetes tests and other lab tests from local US labs can be ordered online from Walk-In-Lab. No doctor's orders are needed. Order, visit the local lab nearest you, and take the tests. The results are available online after a couple of days. A1c, Plasma (Serum) Glucose Test, Two Hour Glucose Tolerance Test, Urine Test, CMP and many other tests are available. For more information go to:

www.reversediabetes101.com/11

Random Glucose Test

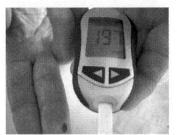

This test is also known as the Fingerstick Capillary Glucose Test. This is a random "snapshot" test of your blood sugar using a glucose meter. Glucose meters are also called glucometers.

Capillaries are the smallest blood vessels in the body. This test is done by using a small lancing device to prick the tip of a finger to obtain a small sample of capillary blood. This drop of blood is placed on a disposable strip in the glucometer. After a few seconds, the test results are shown.

If other symptoms are present, any test that is over 200 mg/dl indicates diabetes. The diagnosis of diabetes should be verified by a health care provider using one or more of the other types of lab tests.

Smart Glucose Meter with Free Phone App

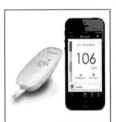

The iHealth Diabetes meter is an inexpensive, compact, blood glucose meter that has a free app that works with Android and Apple smart phones. It provides tests in 5 seconds and simultaneously syncs with your phone. You can share your information with your health care providers and others. This a useful tool to measure your progress in controlling your blood sugar. It can also help you be more accountable to others who can encourage you to achieve your goals. Scroll down to the bottom of the page at the following link for the special bundle price and free shipping.

http://reversediabetes101.com/10

Caring for Type 2 Diabetes

Diet Changes and Exercise Complement Medical Care

Diet and exercise lifestyle changes have been proven to reverse type 2 diabetes and prediabetes. These changes will often eliminate the need for drugs to control the disease.

If you have prediabetes, diet and exercise changes can keep you from developing type 2 diabetes. If you already have diabetes, you should keep your diabetes symptoms under control with the help of medical professionals. You should use diabetes drugs and insulin injections as necessary to get immediate control of your blood sugar levels.

Making changes in diet and exercise habits that can reverse diabetes should not be your only method of treatment. Until you see the results from your lifestyle changes, you need to keep your blood sugar levels under control with the help of a doctor. This will help you avoid dangerous complications of the disease.

Diet changes and exercise are important for reversing type 2 diabetes. Exercise and diet will complement the necessary medical treatment that helps you get immediate control of your blood sugar levels.

Diabetes Medical Treatment

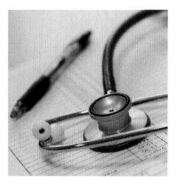

If you have Diabetes, your Doctor will start treatment immediately to lower your blood sugar levels. This is important to slow down or prevent further damage to your body's cells caused by high blood sugar levels.

The following chart shows the number of adults who are being treated in the US for diabetes. It also shows the percentage of the types of treatments they are using to control their blood sugar levels.

US Treatment of Diabetes among People Aged 18 Years or Older with Diagnosed Diabetes

	Number of adults using diabetes medication (millions)	Percentage using diabetes medication (*unadjusted)
Insulin only	2.9	14.0
Both insulin and oral medication	3.1	14.7
Oral medication only	11.9	56.9
Neither insulin nor oral medication	3.0	14.4

*Does not add up to the total number of adults with diagnosed diabetes because of different data sources and methods used. Source: 2010-2012 National Health Interview Survey.

The Importance of Eye and Foot Exams

If a doctor diagnoses you with diabetes, you should see an eye doctor to have a dilated eye exam. This exam checks to see if there is damage to the blood vessels in your eyes caused by diabetes. This exam can help prevent further eye complications and blindness. Diabetes is the leading cause of blindness in adults.

Your doctor should also conduct a foot exam to see if the nerves in your feet are damaged. This nerve damage can produce numbness in your feet. This damage is called neuropathy. It is most often first noticed in the feet. Neuropathy can also affect the hands and other areas of your body. You may be referred to a foot doctor for treatment if you have developed complications in your feet.

10 Important Tests and Exams for Managing Diabetes

These tests and exams are important if you have been diagnosed with Diabetes. These tests may be performed once a year during a routine annual physical exam or more often if needed.

1. **A1c Blood Sugar Test.** This lab test should be done every 3 to 6 months. It is different from blood testing you do yourself. The A1c tells what your blood sugar levels have been during the last three or four months.

2. **Blood Pressure Test.** Hypertension or high blood pressure is common with patients with type 2 diabetes and should be monitored and controlled to prevent additional complications.

3. **Lipid Blood Test.** This test measures different kinds of fats in your blood. This is the test used to measure the "good" cholesterol, "bad" cholesterol and triglycerides.

4. **Dilated Eye Exam.** This exam checks to see if the small blood vessels in your eyes are healthy.

5. **Urine Test.** This checks the amount of protein in your urine to see if your kidneys are healthy.

6. **Complete Foot Exam.** This exam checks to see if the blood circulation, nerves and skin in your feet are healthy. This exam may be performed at every visit to your health care provider.

7. **Mouth Exam.** This exam is useful to determine if you have any complications from diabetes to your gums and teeth

8. **Weight.** Regular weight checks are part of every visit to you doctor, but they should be done more often at home. This will help you monitor your progress towards your weight loss goals.

9. **Flu Shot.** This is a good preventive practice that should be done every fall before flu season. Diabetics are often at greater risk for catching the flu. The flu can cause additional complications and

mess up your blood sugar control. You can avoid this by receiving an annual flu shot from your health care provider.

10. **Pneumococcal Vaccination**. This is also another good preventative practice to avoid several types of serious pneumococcal infections. This vaccination usually lasts 5 to 10 years. You should ask your health care professional if you need it during your next exam.

What Happens if I Ignore My Diabetes?

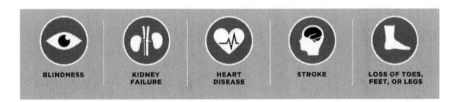

Ignoring diabetes and high blood sugar levels is not going to make the disease go away. If you bury your head in the sand and pretend that your diabetes does not exist, you will severely regret it later.

Uncontrolled high blood sugar levels will end up affecting every part of your body. Your heart, blood vessels, eyes, kidneys, gums and teeth, nerves and your other senses will be affected. One serious complication of uncontrolled high or low blood sugar is a diabetic coma. This dangerous condition sometimes leads to death. You can avoid this, and other serious complications, by taking action to control your blood sugar levels.

Blindness and Eye Problems

Did you know that diabetes is the leading cause of vision loss and blindness among adults? Uncontrolled diabetes can lead to eye problems like diabetic retinopathy. This causes the vision to become blurred with dark patches. Diabetes can cause macular degeneration. This eye disease causes you to be blind in the center of your visual field. Other eye problems include glaucoma and cataracts. You need to have a good action plan to control your blood sugar to avoid devastating eye complications.

Many people have gone blind because they ignored their diabetes. You need to make sure you do not become one of them.

Kidney Related Problems

Diabetes is also the leading cause of kidney failure in the United States of America. Diabetes is listed as the primary cause of kidney failure in 44% of all new cases. In 2011 over 200,000 people in the US were living with kidney failure due to diabetes. Kidney failure causes you to need constant kidney dialysis or a kidney transplant to stay alive.

Heart Disease, Circulatory Problems and Strokes

High blood sugar levels damage blood vessels. This damage can lead to heart and circulatory problems. Most of the people suffering from diabetes also end up suffering from heart disease and high blood pressure.

Uncontrolled diabetes can lead to blood clots in the brain. These can cause strokes. Damaged blood vessels can also cause sexual dysfunction in men. Keeping your diabetes under control lowers your risk for heart disease, strokes and circulatory problems.

Nerve Damage and Amputations

High blood sugar levels in the body can result in severe damage to the nerves. This is diabetic neuropathy. This nerve damage can lead to amputations in the legs and feet. Research also shows that about 60% of non-traumatic lower-limb amputations among people who are over 20 years old occur in people with diagnosed diabetes.

Teeth and Gum Related Problems

Uncontrolled diabetes is usually accompanied by teeth and gum diseases. If you are a diabetic, then regular checkups of your gums and teeth is a must. Untreated teeth and gum conditions can cause tooth loss and other problems that affect your health.

Hyperglycemia and Hypoglycemia

Here is an easy trick to remember the difference between words beginning with "hyper" and "hypo." "Hyper" means "higher" than normal. "Hyper" and "higher" both have the letter "e" in them. "Hypo" means "lower" than normal. "Hypo" and "lower" both have the letter "o" in them.

Hyperglycemia is a result of uncontrolled diabetes. In this condition, the person has extremely high glucose levels that can go as high as 600 mg/dl. High blood sugar levels can result in severe consequences and lead to many additional complications. One of the most life-threating complications of hyperglycemia is a diabetic coma. A diabetic coma could lead to death. High blood sugar levels need prompt medical attention to avoid immediate problems and avoid long-term complications.

The name for low blood sugar is hypoglycemia. A hypoglycemic condition occurs when the blood sugar levels go as low as 60 mg/dl. Low blood sugar occurs if a person has not been eating meals on time or has other health conditions like kidney failure. Hypoglycemic conditions are sometimes caused by diabetes medicines and insulin.

Low blood sugar can cause symptoms of confusion, palpitations, sweating, nausea, dizziness and fainting. Under these circumstances, the person should be given juice or candy immediately to bring the sugar level back to normal.

Low blood sugar can be life threatening if not controlled. In severe cases of low blood sugar, the brain is unable to receive an adequate supply of energy from glucose. A diabetic coma can occur from too little sugar (glucose) in the blood.

If you are taking diabetes medicines or insulin, it is important not to ignore your blood sugar levels. You do not need to let your blood sugar get out of control and be too high or too low. You should regularly check your blood sugar levels, and you should take immediate action to correct any problems before they can cause serious damage to your body.

Increased Medical Costs and Lower Quality of Life

The medical cost for diabetics is usually twice that of non-diabetics. Insulin injections and other medications are expensive. If complications are involved to your eyes, kidneys or feet, the cost can be even higher. If you consider the cost of lost productivity and quality of life issues, the cost can be incalculably higher for diabetics and their families.

Death

Diabetes is the seventh leading cause of deaths in the United States. Diabetes is also a factor in many deaths from heart disease and strokes.

Uncontrolled diabetes is a dangerous condition. Your risk of death from diabetes goes down significantly when you control your blood sugar levels. Controlling your blood sugar allows you to live longer than those who ignore their diabetes. Most people who control their blood sugar levels can live near-normal lives.

There are many problems associated with uncontrolled diabetes. Knowing the consequences of the disease should help you to understand how it would be much better for you to control your blood sugar levels. It is OK to take medicines to make this happen if you are already in trouble with high blood sugar. Medicines and insulin will solve your problems temporarily. However, if you will learn to control or reverse your type 2 diabetes symptoms without drugs by making changes in your diet and exercise habits, you will be much better off in the long run

.

Step 2: Discover Diabetes Reversal Solutions

Can Type 2 Diabetes Be Reversed?

The short answer is, yes. Type 2 diabetes is reversible. There is evidence that two methods have been successful in reversing diabetes. Doctors have studied very low-calorie, low-carb diets and determined that most people within 10 years of the onset of type 2 diabetes can reverse their symptoms in a few weeks. Weight-loss surgery also produces the side effect of type 2 diabetes reversal soon after surgery. This fact has been known for at least 20 years. Yes, it is possible to reverse type 2 diabetes and not have to take medicines or insulin. There is real medical evidence that verifies this fact.

What Is Type 2 Diabetes Reversal?

Diabetes reversal and diabetes remission mean the same thing. If you have type 2 diabetes, remission or reversal means you no longer have to take drugs or insulin to manage your diabetes. You are asymptomatic for diabetes. In other words, you no longer have any symptom of the disease, your lab tests show normal results, and your blood sugar levels are under control. If you have normal test results, no symptoms of diabetes, and if you are not taking any medications for diabetes, your diabetes is reversed.

Most doctors agree diabetes is in remission if the symptoms subside for a year or longer. Remission does not mean that diabetes is cured. Remission means the symptoms of diabetes have disappeared and medicines or insulin are no longer needed. Just as cancer can go into successful remission with treatment, diabetes can also go into successful remission.

Since 90% or more of diagnosed diabetes is type 2 diabetes, it is good news that this type of diabetes can be reversed under the right conditions. However, the desire to achieve diabetes reversal comes with one big catch—it takes motivation and determination to eat less, lose weight and keep the weight off.

Can Very Low-Calorie, Low Carb Diets Reverse Type 2 Diabetes?

Professor Roy Taylor from Newcastle University, UK documented the success of very low-calorie, low-carb diets to reverse type 2 diabetes. He reported his findings in an article in the American Diabetes Association journal *Diabetes Care* in May 2016*.

> *Professor Roy Taylor said, "What we have shown is that it is possible to reverse your diabetes, even if you have had the condition for a long time, up to around 10 years. If you have had the diagnosis for longer than that, then do not give up hope—major improvement in blood sugar control is possible.*

Professor Taylor reported that a 600-800-calorie daily diet consisting of three high-protein shakes and 8 ounces (240 g) of fresh vegetables reversed diabetes in 8 weeks. This diet was the most successful on patients who had type 2 diabetes less than 10 years.

The 30 study participants had diabetes from 6 months to 23 years. The research was able to determine in advance if participants could reverse their diabetes by determining if their pancreas was still producing some insulin. Twelve participants in the study, who had type 2 diabetes less than 10 years, reversed their diabetes. Participants in the study lost an average of 31 pounds (14 kg), but they still remained overweight or obese at the end of the study. After 6 months, the diabetes reversal was still intact.

70% of severely obese people do not have diabetes. Professor Taylor said:

> *This supports our theory of a Personal Fat Threshold. If a person gains more weight than they personally can tolerate, then diabetes is triggered, but if they then lose that amount of weight then they go back to normal.*

The evidence is growing that fat build up inside the liver and pancreas can be reduced quickly with very low-calorie, low-carb diets. This fat decrease may be what reverses type 2 diabetes. Fat loss inside the pancreas may be what unclogs the pancreas and returns insulin production to normal.

This 2016 study was a longer follow-up study to the one in 2011 that found type 2 diabetes was reversible with a very low-calorie, low-carb diet. A larger study with 230 participants is now underway. This new study hopes to prove the results are duplicable with other doctors and nurses using the same methods.

Diabetes Care 2016 May, Roy Taylor, et al.
Very Low Calorie Diet and 6 Months Weight Stability
http://dx.doi.org/10.2337/dc15-1942

Diabetes Care 2013 Apr, Roy Taylor
Reversal of Type 2 Diabetes by Bariatric Surgery or Hypocaloric Diet
http://dx.doi.org/10.2337/dc12-1805

Diabetology 2011 June, Roy Taylor, et al.
Reversal of Type 2 Diabetes
http://link.springer.com/article/10.1007/s00125-011-2204-7

Can Weight-Loss Surgery Reverse Type 2 Diabetes?

There is a term that describes people who are 100 pounds or more over their ideal body weight. The term for this is morbid obesity or extreme obesity.

> *One of the definitions of "morbid" means*
> *to have an abnormal interest in dying.*

Extreme obesity causes people to have many health problems. Extreme obesity causes loss of quality of life, and in some cases, premature death. Extreme obesity can shorten people's lives. Extreme obesity costs individuals and society billions of dollars each year.

In the US approximately 5% of the population is considered extremely obese. This means millions of people in the US and millions more around the world are extremely overweight. The problem has increased over the years and shows no signs of letting up anytime soon.

Doctors have developed drastic weight loss surgical procedures to help those who are extremely obese. This type of surgery is bariatric surgery or weight-loss surgery. Bariatric surgery is a last resort surgery. These surgeries are performed on people who are extremely obese and suffering from life-threatening problems like diabetes and high blood pressure.

> *It has been known for over 20 years that many extremely obese patients who have weight-loss surgery have their type 2 diabetes go into remission or reversal. This is a common side effect of weight-loss surgery.*

With a large number of gastric bypass surgeries, diabetes reversal takes place within a few days. Diabetes reversal occurred before the patient experienced any weight loss from the surgery. The scientific reasons behind this are unclear, but the fact remains type 2 diabetes is reversible.

A curious fact is that the type of bariatric surgery affects the diabetes reversal rates. Bariatric bypass surgery patients taking insulin had twice as many diabetes reversals than patients undergoing laparoscopic banding (62% vs. 29.5 %). Similar diabetes reversal rates were observed in surgery patients only taking oral medications.

Bariatric surgery is a very effective method of weight loss for many extremely obese people. Nevertheless, bariatric surgery, with its risk and complications, should only be used as a last resort to save the lives of extremely obese patients. One good takeaway from bariatric surgery is it confirms long-term diabetes reversal is possible under the right conditions.

Bariatric bypass surgery demonstrates that weight loss alone is not the only factor in type 2 diabetes reversal. Further scientific study is necessary, and hopefully, researchers will soon discover the reasons why bariatric surgery causes type 2 diabetes reversal.

Diabetes Care 2015 April, Ali Tavakkoli, et al.
Diabetes Remission after Bariatric Surgery
http://dx.doi.org/10.2337/dc14-1751

Diabetes Care 2013 August, Sangeeta R. Kashyap.
Metabolic Effects of Bariatric Surgery and Diabetes
http://dx.doi.org/10.2337/dc12-1596

Lessons Learned from Weight-loss surgery

While these surgical procedures for those who are extremely obese can help them lose one-half their body weight or more, these surgeries do not come without risks. There are many possible complications and side effects. Lifetime lifestyle changes are necessary to avoid side effects for anyone who has undergone weight-loss surgery. Having one's stomach bypassed or reduced by up to 90% changes the way the body absorbs food.

After the surgery, weight-loss surgery patients are given a strict diet plan. They must eat differently and exercise to continue to lose weight and reach their weight loss goals. Bariatric patients must take vitamins the rest of their lives. This is necessary to supplement the loss of nutrient absorption resulting from surgically eliminating parts of their digestive system.

About 20%-30% of all bariatric surgery patients do not meet their weight loss goals, and their surgeries are considered failures. Weight-loss surgery patients must eat less to insure the desired long-term results of the surgery. If a weight-loss surgery patient does not change their eating habits, they will not see any weight loss after their surgery.

> *Successful bariatric surgeries are successful because the patients changed their eating habits and followed the post-surgery rules. They followed strict diet plans. This is what made them lose weight and keep it off. After the surgery, they ate substantially less and lost weight quickly.*

Unfortunately, some weight loss patients have other issues that they must deal with mentally before they can eat less and lose weight. Many times extremely obese people have emotional barriers to weight loss. After the surgery, they continue to overeat and do not lose weight. For these individuals, psychological counseling is necessary to help them change their eating behavior to reach their goals.

The transformation of eating habits and exercise patterns by one's own self-control is the key to weight loss by surgical methods or any other methods. This type of weight loss can be maintained indefinitely.

Weight-loss surgery can be useful to some extremely obese individuals as a way to surgically induce the self-control they need to help them to lose weight. However, weight-loss surgery should not be seen as a miracle cure-all for weight loss. Self-control without surgery should be considered the miracle most people need to lose weight.

> *Weight loss by self-control comes without the lifetime*
> *complications and adverse side effects of having parts of*
> *your stomach and intestines surgically altered.*

Weight loss methods, surgical or otherwise, do not come without a cost in effort, motivation and determination. Weight loss from self-control is better than surgery for most overweight people who are not extremely obese.

Learning what to eat and how to eat can be just as effective as weight-loss surgery. However, this knowledge will not work unless the person alters their eating behavior and makes lifestyle changes.

Weight-loss surgery is not the answer for most overweight people. Weight loss using very low-calorie, low-carb diets, along with exercise, remains the best bet for most people who want to lose weight to reverse type 2 diabetes.

Essential Nutrition

Every day you make choices about what you eat and drink. A basic understanding of nutrition is essential for eating an optimal diet to control and reverse type 2 diabetes. This essential nutrition information forms the backbone for a healthy eating lifestyle. Understanding nutrition is also necessary to understand how to eat differently to burn fat. Fat-burning diets do work and can be useful to lose weight quickly.

Changes in what you eat can often be hard because old eating habits are hard to break. New habits can be made, and you will begin seeing results in the way you feel and look sooner than you might think. Just make up your mind to develop new habits and then put forth the effort and be determined to change. Do not over think it. Just do it.

Carbs

What is a carb? Carb is short for carbohydrate. Carbohydrates are molecules that are made up of carbon, oxygen and hydrogen. Carbohydrates are used by the body as its mains source of energy. Sugars and starches are carbohydrates. Glucose is the main form of sugar used by your brain and muscles. Starches and sugars are converted into the simple sugar glucose and then used for body functions, movement or fat storage.

Glycemic Index

The term "glycemic" means causing glucose (sugar) to enter in the blood. In 1981, a scientist at the University of Toronto, David Jenkins, invented the Glycemic Index. It measures how fast blood sugar levels rise after eating different types of carbohydrates. Carbohydrates are made up of different types of starches and sugars that raise the blood sugar (glucose levels) in the blood.

> *Many references use the abbreviation of GI to refer to Glycemic Index.*

Lower Glycemic Index foods take longer to cause blood sugar to rise. High Glycemic Index foods take a shorter time raise blood sugar levels. Controlling the spikes of high blood sugar and overall blood sugar levels are important goals for everyone with diabetes. The Glycemic Index ranges from a low of 1 to a high of 100. The Glycemic Index is 100 for glucose, 86 for mashed potatoes and 32 for strawberries.

Helpful Tip: High glycemic foods should be avoided.
Foods made with white refined sugar or white flour tend to
have high glycemic values. You should avoid any bread,
cakes or sweets made with white sugar and white flour.
You should also avoid most processed foods and breakfast
cereal with added sugar. Read the labels and put it back
on the shelf if it contains added sugar.

When sugar from food takes longer to enter the bloodstream, it has more time to be used for energy. Foods that raise your blood sugar quickly will cause your body to store this energy as fat. Foods that take longer to convert to sugar may also lower your insulin resistance, which is a major underlying cause of type 2 diabetes. Foods that raise blood sugar quickly will cause you to feel hungry sooner than foods that take longer to digest.

The Glycemic Index has been divided into 3 categories: Low, Medium and High. This is the Glycemic Ranking used by most diets.

Most Popular Glycemic Index Ranking	
High	70 and greater
Medium	56 to 69
Low	55 and less

This index ranking has probably been influenced by the food industry to include more foods in the lower range. This might not be that beneficial for anyone trying to control blood sugar levels. A better Glycemic Index ranking is this one below. If your goal is to control your blood sugar levels, this alternative Glycemic Index Ranking is more useful.

Alternative Diabetes Glycemic Index Ranking	
High	50 and greater
Medium	36 to 50
Low	35 and less

The lower range is 35 and below. Foods in this range provide the maximum time for blood sugar levels to rise. Lower Glycemic Index foods are better for managing your blood sugar levels and for avoiding blood sugar spikes. High Glycemic Index foods with high levels of sugar or high fructose corn syrup spike your blood sugar levels almost immediately. All sugary soft drinks fit into this category.

You should try to eat as many foods that are 35 or below in the Glycemic Index. You should also eat fewer foods that are higher than 35.

The University of Sydney in Australia has a website with tons of valuable information on the Glycemic Index.

www.glycemicindex.com

On the first page, there is a handy little search box that lets you type in the food name or a range of glycemic values. For example, a search for foods with a Glycemic Index less than 35 yielded over 500 results.

Glycemic Index of Common Foods

Category	Food	Index*
Beans	Soy	14
	Red lentils	27
	Kidney	33
Bread	Sprouted Grain Bread (Ezekiel Bread)	36
	Pumpernickel	49
	White	69
	Whole wheat	72
Cereals	All bran	54
	Corn flakes	83
	Oatmeal	53
	Puffed rice	90
	Shredded wheat	70
Dairy	Milk, ice cream, yogurt	34–38
Fruit	Strawberries	32
	Apples	38
	Oranges	43
	Orange juice	49
	Bananas	61
Grains	Barley	22
	Brown rice	66
	White rice	72
Pasta	—	38
Potatoes	Sweet	50

	Mashed (white)	72
	Instant mashed (white)	86
Snacks	Potato chips	56
	Oatmeal cookies	57
	Corn chips	72
Sugar	Fructose (fruit sugar- not high fructose)	22
	Refined sugar	64
	High Fructose Corn Sugar	68
	Honey	91
	Glucose	100

*Note: The Glycemic Index Values in preceding table may vary slightly depending on testing conditions. The method of cooking or preparing food can also make a difference. Other conditions may also vary. An underripe banana may have a Glycemic Index value of 30 and a ripe banana might have a value of 60.

Fiber

Fiber is considered a carbohydrate, but it does not raise blood sugar levels. In fact, fiber slows down the digestion of other carbohydrates. This helps to slow down the rise of blood sugar levels and avoid blood sugar spikes.

Fiber is the part of vegetables, beans and grains that pass through the digestive system undigested. Fiber is best known for preventing constipation. Fiber also has other benefits such as helping to maintain a healthy weight and lowering your risk of diabetes and heart disease. There are several positive health benefits to be gained from eating a variety of high fiber natural foods.

Fiber can be classified into two categories: soluble fiber and insoluble fiber. Most plant-based food like beans and oatmeal contain both soluble and insoluble fiber.

Soluble Fiber. Soluble fiber dissolves in water and forms a gel-like substance. Soluble fiber helps to lower cholesterol and glucose levels. Soluble fiber is found in oats, beans, peas, carrots, psyllium, apples and citrus fruits.

Insoluble Fiber. Insoluble fiber helps move materials through the digestive tract, normalizes bowel movements and relieves constipation. Wheat bran, whole-wheat flour, nuts, beans and vegetables like green beans and cauliflower are good sources of insoluble fiber.

Proteins

Proteins are organic molecules that are made of the basic elements of carbon, hydrogen, oxygen nitrogen and sulfur. The basic elements form interlinked chains of amino acids that are the building blocks for the basic cell structures of the body. Proteins form muscles, tissues, blood components and perform many other essential functions.

Protein from animal sources can deliver all the protein you need. These sources include meat and dairy products. Animal sources of protein contain all the necessary amino acids required by the body. Other valuable sources of protein include vegetarian sources such as fruits, vegetables, grains, nuts and seeds. Vegetable sources of protein usually lack one or more of the necessary essential amino acids. This deficiency can be made up by combining various sources of vegetarian proteins such as rice and beans. Rice and beans together contain all the necessary essential amino acids.

Proteins can be used for energy. The amino acids in proteins can be converted to carbohydrates by removing the nitrogen molecule. Carbohydrate molecules are easily broken down into glucose. Proteins are long complex molecules and may take more than three hours to digest.

Water

Water is essential for life. It is very important to body functions including digestion and elimination. Water can aid in weight loss because it provides hydration and it is calorie free. Drinking water before meals also helps you feel full and this helps you eat less. Drinking water before meals and throughout the day can help you lose weight and keep it off.

Your age, weight and activity level determine the amount of water you need. It is recommended that women drink at least 11 cups (91 ounces) and men drink at least 15 cups (125 ounces) of water per day.

Vitamins

Vitamins are vital organic nutrients created by living organisms that the body must have to maintain itself. They are important to functions such as immunity and metabolism. Vitamins are absorbed by the walls of the intestines during digestion. Vitamins come in two broad groups: water-soluble and fat-soluble.

Water-Soluble Vitamins. Water-soluble vitamins can be dissolved in water. Water-soluble vitamins are the B vitamins and Vitamin C. Water-soluble vitamins are also easily destroyed by cooking. Vegetables should be steamed or cooked at low temperature or eaten raw to preserve the water-soluble vitamins. Water-soluble vitamins are not stored in the body and are obtained from supplements are food. After breaking down the vitamins during digestion, the body takes what it needs and excretes the excess from the body.

Fat-Soluble Vitamins. Fat-soluble vitamins are dissolved by fat. Fat-soluble vitamins need fat in order to be absorbed. The fat-soluble vitamins are A, D, K and E. Fat-soluble vitamins are stored in the liver and body fat for use when needed. If fat-soluble vitamins are ingested in large amounts, they can build up to toxic levels.

Water-Soluble Vitamins	Fat-Soluble Vitamins
Thiamin	A
Riboflavin	D
Niacin	K
B6	E
B12	
Biotin	
Folic Acid	
Pantothenic Acid	
Vitamin C	

Minerals

Minerals are found naturally in water, rocks and soil. Minerals are not made by living organisms and they are called inorganic. Vitamins are manufactured by living organisms such as plants and animals and are considered organic. Organic and inorganic substances are science terms. You must have inorganic and organic substances to live. They are necessary foundation blocks for life.

Organic and inorganic terms have nothing to do with food labeled "organic food" in grocery stores. Food labeled "organic food" refers to how the food was grown. "Organic food" in stores actually contains both organic and inorganic substances.

In science terms, plants and animals make organic substance. Inorganic substances are minerals and other chemicals found in the earth and air.

Doctors usually have routine blood tests performed to check the level of inorganic minerals in your body. This helps them determine the balance of minerals found in your blood. This can tell them many things including the health of your liver and kidneys. These lab tests are called Basic Metabolic Panels (BMP) and Comprehensive Metabolic Panels (CMP).

Na – Sodium. Sodium is found in common table salt. It is the first half of the chemical combination of salt which sodium and chloride (NaCl). Most people get plenty of sodium in their diets. Some people need to cut back their salt intake. Sodium is an important electrolyte found in the body. Electrolytes are necessary to conduct electricity in the body. Electrolytes are essential for maintaining the proper balance of fluids between the inside and outside of cells. This is important for proper hydration, muscle function and nerve impulses.

Cl - Chloride. Chloride is part of the chemical makeup of salt. It is the is the Cl in NaCl (sodium chloride). Elemental chlorine by itself is a gas that is dangerous because it rapidly combines with other elements. When bound to other elements like sodium, the Na in NaCl (sodium chloride), it is safe. Chloride is a mineral substance and chlorine is a gas. Chlorine is used to purify drinking water and in cleaning products because it is deadly to bacteria. Chloride is a necessary mineral for life and is obtained from salt. It is an essential element in bodily fluids and digestive juices. It helps regulate the body's chemical balances. It is also found in sports drinks along with other mineral electrolytes of sodium, potassium, magnesium and calcium.

K– Potassium. Potassium helps regulate the movement of fluids, nutrients and waste from your cells. A lack of potassium can lead to high blood pressure and cause you to be irritable.

Ca – Calcium. Calcium is the basic building block for strong bones and teeth. It also plays an important part in the chemistry of muscles and other tissues in the body.

Mg – Magnesium. Magnesium is necessary for a healthy heartbeat and strong bones. It is also involved in over 300 chemical reactions in the body.

P – Phosphorous. Phosphorous is important for bone health and is necessary to provide energy to cells.

S – Sulfur. The body needs sulfur to make hair, cartilage, skin and nails. It is also necessary for proper nervous system function.

Trace Minerals

Trace minerals are valuable to maintain a healthy body. The quantities of trace minerals that are required are far less than the major minerals.

Trace minerals include copper, zinc, iron, iodine, manganese, fluoride, molybdenum, selenium and chromium. Most of these trace minerals are found in enzymes or hormones required in metabolism. Other trace minerals such as arsenic, boron, cobalt nickel, silicon, vanadium and cobalt may or may not be necessary for the body. Trace minerals are toxic at high levels. Some trace minerals like arsenic, nickel and chromium may even cause cancer.

Fats and Oils

Fats come in two main varieties: saturated and unsaturated. Unsaturated fats are liquid at room temperature and saturated fats are solid at room temperature. Butter, lard and coconut oil are saturated fats. Olive oil and other liquid vegetable oils are unsaturated fats. Saturated and unsaturated fats that are plant derived are the best type of oils and fat you can eat.

Saturated Fats. Saturated fats found in animal foods been linked to heart disease. Animal fat intake should be limited. Not all saturated fats are bad. Plant-derived saturated fats like coconut oil have proven to be beneficial.

Unsaturated Fats. Unsaturated fats are the oils taken from plants. Olive oil and other vegetable oils, nuts and seeds all contain unsaturated fats.

Cold pressed vegetable oils are made without the use of heat. Cold pressed oils retain their nutritional ingredients when they are processed. Cold pressed extra-virgin oils are considered the best oils to use regularly for salads and low-temperature cooking.

Cooking oils are not cold pressed. They are heated, refined, bleached and deodorized during processing. This type of processing damages or destroys most of the nutritional ingredients, but these oils tolerate higher temperature cooking better.

There are two types of unsaturated fats: monounsaturated fats and polyunsaturated fats. These fats promote heart health. The chemical nature of the fats determines if they are monounsaturated or polyunsaturated.

Monounsaturated Fats: Foods that contain monounsaturated fats include:

- olive, oil, sesame oil and canola oil
- peanut butter, peanuts and cashews
- avocados and olives
- sesame seeds

Polyunsaturated Fats. Foods that are high in polyunsaturated fats include:

- sunflower seeds, pumpkin seeds, pine nuts and walnuts
- corn oil, safflower oil and soybean oil

Polyunsaturated Omega-3 Fats. Omega-3 fats are polyunsaturated fats that have been found to aid in heart health. They also help lower cholesterol and triglycerides. Sources of omega-3 fats include:

- salmon, mackerel, herring and tuna
- flax seeds, chia seeds and walnuts

Artificial Trans Fats are the hydrogenated and partially-hydrogenated oils used commercially for preparing fast foods, baked goods, snack foods and margarines. Their purpose is to extend product shelf life and keep oils from becoming rancid. Trans fats are unnatural, manmade substances.

Artificial trans fats are vegetable oils that are processed in a factory and become a new type of oil that is never found in nature. Hydrogenated fats are made by heating up vegetable oils with hydrogen gas in the presence of metal catalysts. This process is called hydrogenation.

In 2015 the Food and Drug Administration (FDA) made a determination that by 2018 food companies should phase out the use of artificial trans-fat oils in food products. You should check all food labels and do not buy or eat anything with partially-hydrogenated or hydrogenated, artificial trans fats.

Artificial trans fats cause even worse health results than saturated fats. Artificial trans fats are linked to increased risks of heart disease, strokes and type 2 diabetes. They cause a rise in bad cholesterol and allow hormones and the nervous system to create chronic inflammation. Chronic inflammation is linked to many serious adverse health effects

If you can reduce chronic inflammation by not eating foods with artificial trans fats, you will feel better, reduce the chance for chronic diseases, improve your immune system and slow the aging process.

According to the FDA, artificial trans fats can be found in many foods. They are usually listed on ingredient labels as hydrogenated oil or partially-hydrogenated oil.

- baked goods (cookies, cakes, pies, and crackers)
- snack foods (potato chips and microwave popcorn)
- fried fast foods (French fries, fried chicken, and doughnuts)
- refrigerated dough products (biscuits, rolls, and frozen pizza)
- vegetable shortening and stick margarine
- coffee creamer

How Fat-Burning, Very Low-Calorie, Low-Carb Diets Work

The Biological Principle of Ketosis

Fat-burning, very low-calorie, low-carb diets work because of the biological principle of ketosis. The body needs energy to survive. During times of starvation, the body burns ketones for energy instead of carbs. The body gets most of these ketones from the energy stored in fat cells. Ketosis is the condition of the body when it is fueled almost entirely by ketones produced from fat burning.

The brain and muscles are designed to use ketones as a substitute for glucose during periods of famine. Fasting and low-calorie, low-carb diets use the principle of ketosis to burn fat. Ketosis is a beneficial biological process that you can use to burn fat rapidly in your body.

Acetone is a normal byproduct of ketosis. Acetone can be smelled on the breath of a person in ketosis. It is described as a sweet, fruity smell or a nail polish smell. Acetone is also eliminated in the urine.

During ketosis, daily activities can be carried on as usual. Many people experience improved mental functioning when they are burning ketones instead of glucose while fasting or consuming a low-calorie, low-carb diet.

When you stop eating carbs, you decrease the amount of glucose stored in the body and you begin to burn fat. Everyone has a 24-hour supply of glucose stored in the muscles and liver in the form of glycogen. On a low calorie, low-carb diet, the glycogen level in the body is lowered and ketones are used for energy. Amino acids from proteins also contribute to energy, but after two or three days, Ketones from fat become the main source of energy.

On a low-calorie, low-carb diet plan, you must limit carbohydrates. You should eliminate starchy foods and foods refined sugar or high fructose corn syrup. You should eat less than 60 grams of carbs per day to stay in ketosis. This limits you to non-starchy vegetables and maybe a few berries.

You should also restrict the amount of calories you eat from fats and oils. You should consume some protein, but not so much that you increase your total calories beyond your daily limit. The amino acids in protein can be converted to glucose and can stop ketosis if too much is consumed.

Diets do not work for most people because they do not stay on the diets for very long. They never enter into a state of ketosis. They quit the diets before they see any results. Nevertheless, there is a lot of evidence that low-calorie, low-carb diets are effective for weight loss when followed for a few weeks. Strictly following these diets for will keep you in ketosis.

Fasting for a limited time, or going on a low-calorie, low-carbohydrate diet will create the conditions for fat-burning ketosis. Ketosis can help you lose weight and control your blood sugar levels. It also has several other benefits like lowering blood pressure, triglycerides and cholesterol.

If you can stay on a low-carb, low-calorie, you can achieve significant results in a few weeks. The principle of ketosis fat burning is a sound principle for weight loss. The major drawback is that it requires a drastic change in diet for a few weeks to obtain the desired results.

Ketosis vs. Ketoacidosis

Fat-burning ketosis is good, but ketoacidosis is a dangerous condition. Type 1 Diabetes often causes ketoacidosis. This is why another name for ketoacidosis is Diabetic Ketoacidosis (DKA). DKA does sometimes occur in Type 2 diabetes when the pancreas does not produce insulin. It occurs rarely in people without diabetes.

Ketosis and ketoacidosis are two different conditions and should not be confused. Ketosis is the way the body produces energy from ketones when glucose is not available. Lower levels of ketones are not dangerous in the body.

In ketoacidosis, a lack of insulin stops glucose from being used for energy. This can cause high levels of ketones in the blood from ketosis. When the ketones build up faster than they can be burned for energy, they cause the body chemistry to be overly acidic. Ketoacidosis does not occur in healthy people or diabetics who are controlling their blood sugar levels.

The levels of ketones in the blood determine the condition of ketosis in the body. Ketosis is not dangerous when ketones are used for energy and diabetes is controlled. Keeping blood sugar levels in a normal range will prevent ketoacidosis.

Excessive thirst and the need to urinate often are symptoms of high ketone levels. Belly pain, nausea, tiredness, confusion and having trouble breathing are also severe symptoms of ketoacidosis. Anyone experiencing these symptoms needs to seek immediate medical attention.

Urine test strips, as well as ketone meters, are available to test ketone levels. Ketone meters are more accurate than test strips, but they are more expensive.

The following chart shows the level ketones that indicate the condition of ketosis in the body.

Ketone Urine Test Results

Blood Concentration (millimolar)	KetosisCondition
< 0.2	not in ketosis
0.2 - 0.5	slight/mild ketosis
0.5 - 3.0	induced/nutritional ketosis
2.5 - 3.5	post-exercise ketosis
3.0 - 6.0	starvation ketosis
15 - 25	ketoacidosis

Ketones are a natural source of energy for the body. Ketosis is good for weight loss and is an important principle for type 2 diabetes reversal.

What Are Calories?

The energy stored up in carbohydrates and fat cells is measured in units called kilocalories.

> *One kilocalorie is a science word that represents the amount of energy it takes to raise the temperature of a kilogram (2.2 pounds) of water one degree Celsius.*

The amount of energy in a kilocalorie forms the basis for calculating how much energy is in the food we eat. Food label calories are actually scientific units of kilocalories. For our purposes in this book, calories mean food label calories.

Calories in Foods and Drinks	
Proteins (meat/ eggs/cheese)	4 calories per gram
Carbohydrates (grains/starches)	4 calories per gram
Ethanol (alcohol in drinks)	7 calories per gram
Fats (oils/butter/fat)	9 calories per gram

Why is it important to know how much energy is in a calorie of food? This knowledge simplifies the concept of exercise, dieting and weight loss.

When you know how many calories of energy are in the food you are eating, you can design a diet based on the number calories of energy you need to eat in order to lose weight. The fewer calories you eat, the faster you will lose weight.

When you know how many calories of energy are stored in a pound of fat, you can understand how many calories of energy you must use to lose weight. The more calories you burn in exercise, the faster you will lose weight.

Exercise and Weight Loss

The Simple Math behind Weight Gain and Weight Loss

You need energy to live. Your main source of energy comes from the food you eat. When you eat less energy than required, you lose weight. If you eat more food than is required for daily activities, you gain weight. The math behind this is simple.

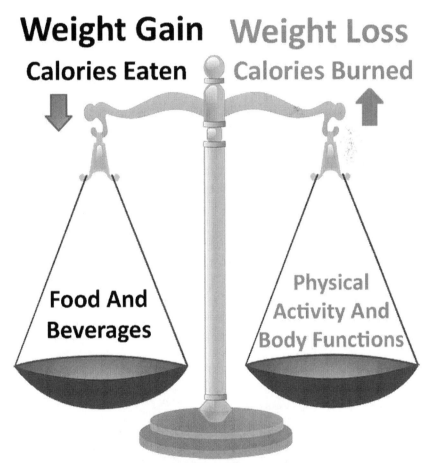

Calories Eaten = Calories Burned = No Weight Loss or Gain
More Food Eaten than Needed For Physical Actvities = Weight Gain
Less Food Eaten than Needed For Physical Actvities = Weight Loss

The previous description of weight loss is a bit of an oversimplification of the process. How the human body stores and uses energy is more complex than this, but it illustrates the point— fat stores build up when you eat more than you need. If you can eat less than you need for your body functions and physical activities, you will burn up your fat storage and lose weight. This is the simple math behind weight gain and weight loss. Admittedly, this is easier said than done for most people.

The math required to lose weight may be simple, but the problem is applying this math to your lifestyle. If diabetes is linked to inactivity and excess consumption of food, then the solution will be found in doing the opposite. To lose weight, you need to eat less and move more.

How Much Exercise Does It Take to Burn One Pound of Fat?

Nutrition Facts

12 servings per container

Serving size   1/2 muffin (114g)

	Per 1/2 muffin		Per 1 muffin	
Calories	**380**		**760**	
		% DV*		**% DV***
Total Fat	16g	**21%**	32g	**41%**
Saturated Fat	3g	**15%**	6g	**30%**
Trans Fat	0g		0g	
Cholesterol	50mg	**17%**	100mg	**33%**
Sodium	480mg	**21%**	960mg	**42%**
Total Carb.	56g	**20%**	112g	**41%**
Dietary Fiber	2g	**7%**	4g	**14%**
Total Sugars	32g		64g	
Incl. Added Sugars	30g	**60%**	60g	**120%**
Protein	3g		6g	
Vitamin D	0.1mcg	0%	0.2mcg	2%
Calcium	40mg	4%	80mg	6%
Iron	2mg	10%	4mg	20%
Potassium	190mg	4%	380mg	8%

* The % Daily Value (DV) tells you how much a nutrient in a serving of food contributes to a daily diet. 2,000 calories a day is used for general nutrition advice.

Here is a sample food label for a 114 g muffin. 114 g is about 4 ounces or 1/4 of a pound. This food label says this muffin contains 760 food calories of energy.

There are 3,500 calories of energy stored in one pound of fat. If you eat 5 of these muffins that contain 760 calories each, you will have eaten the number of calories in 1.08 pounds of fat (3,800 calories.)

How much exercise is required to lose one pound of weight if one pound of weight equals 3,500 calories?

Here are some examples that illustrate this point. Keep in mind that running a mile burns up more calories than walking a mile.

A 155-pound runner burns up about 700 calories an hour at a 10-mile per hour pace. After five hours of running, 3,500 calories are burned. This is the same amount of calories in one pound of fat. Unfortunately, runners burn up glucose and glycogen before they burn up fat. Runners will burn up glucose obtained from recent meals along with the glycogen stored in their muscles and liver before their fat storage is used for energy.

This same person walking slowly at 2 miles per hour would only burn up141 calories. To burn up 700 calories that person would have to walk 5 miles. At 2 miles per hour, this would take 2 and 1/2 hours. At this pace, the walker would have to walk for 12 1/2 hours to burn up 3,500 calories. This is the equivalent calories in one pound of fat. Again, walking burns up glucose and glycogen before it burns fat.

Weight loss occurs when your daily activities use up more calories than you take in. Eating less and exercising more is necessary for weight loss. Exercise is important to help you lose weight, but as you can see from this illustration, losing weight by running or walking will not happen overnight. Real weight loss comes from eating fewer 760-calorie muffins and combining that with more exercise.

Regular Exercise Has Many Benefits

Just because you found out it takes a lot of exercise to lose one pound of weight, do not become discouraged. Regular exercise has other benefits that make it worth the time and effort.

> *Many athletes and some ordinary people have experienced a sense of euphoria after running long distances. This does not happen to everyone, but it happens enough that the term "runners high" is used to describe the experience.*

Regular vigorous exercise can increase your metabolism. A person who exercises vigorously will continue to burn more calories during the day than someone who is sedentary. Even if you exercise moderately, the benefits are many. However, if you can vigorously exercise for 45 minutes or more three times a week you will see a greater benefit.

An active runner will continue to receive the benefit of burning more calories for several hours after they stop running In fact, any vigorous exercise for at least 45 minutes seems to cause this effect.

Exercise not only helps the body to burn more fuel, it also helps the brain receive more oxygen. Exercise can improve your mental alertness and mental attitude. Exercise also helps you regulate stress hormones and overcome feelings of anxiety and depression.

It is important to exercise, but the fastest way to lose weight is to exercise and eat less. If you combine moderate or vigorous exercise with consuming fewer calories, you will lose weight. This is a scientific fact.

Here is a link to a commercial-free site that lists the calories in 8,000 different foods and the calories burned during different types of exercises. You will also find free resources to help you lose weight and live healthier:

https://www.supertracker.usda.gov/

10 Guidelines for Blood Sugar Management

Diabetes is a disease that requires the individual to participate in its management. If you have diabetes you are responsible for what you eat and what you do not eat. You are responsible for checking your blood sugar levels and taking your medications. You are also responsible for your level of activity or inactivity.

If you have diabetes, you must make choices daily about what you eat and how much you move. If you take it one day at a time, you can control your blood sugar levels and live a near normal life. The most important changes you need to make in your life are to eat fewer carbs, eat healthier and become more active.

If you have prediabetes, these 10 guidelines will also be valuable to you. They can help you prevent prediabetes from becoming type 2 diabetes.

1. Avoid Unhealthy Carbohydrates and Fats

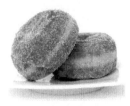

You should avoid foods that are high in refined carbohydrates and starchy foods that provide little if any additional essential nutrients. The carbs in sweets, chocolates, donuts and soft drinks can rapidly increase your blood sugar levels to unhealthy levels.

You should avoid any food made from white sugar, white flour or high fructose corn syrup. Choose natural foods that are not highly processed.

You should avoid meats full of saturated fat or only occasionally eat them. Substitute lean proteins such as fish instead.

You should avoid eating fried foods cooked in vegetable cooking oils. Refined vegetable cooking oils produce harmful chemicals at high temperatures. These chemicals end up in the food. Cook at a lower temperature with unrefined oils like coconut oil or extra-virgin olive oil.

You should avoid any food or snack food that contains artificial trans fats. These ingredients are labeled as hydrogenated or partially-hydrogenated oils. Artificial trans fats should be avoided like plague. They adversely affect the circulatory system and increase inflammation in the body.

2. Select the Right Foods in the Right Amounts

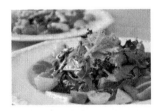

The more fresh vegetables you eat, the better off you will be. Your best food choices will always be fresh vegetables and other fresh foods that have not been refined and processed.

The dietary fiber present in fruits and vegetables plays a significant role in controlling diabetes. It delays the release of glucose into the blood by slowing down the digestive process. In short, a proper diet for a diabetic should include fiber and protein rich foods and few, if any, fatty foods and sugary foods.

If you have diabetes this does not mean you have to eliminate carbohydrates completely from your diet. You just need to realize carbohydrates will raise your blood sugar, and you need to limit the amount that you consume at any one time.

Some fats and oils are considered essential. They are necessary to maintain optimal health and brain function. Remember, fats contain nine calories per gram. This is more than twice as many as the four calories per gram in carbs. Consuming fats and oils can cause you to gain weight faster than eating carbs. It is ok to eat a few essential fats or oils that are necessary for optimal health, but don't overdo eating them. This is especially important if you are trying to lose weight.

Some sources of good carbohydrates are whole grain breads, pastas, whole grain cereals, etc. Check the glycemic value as discussed earlier. Select low glycemic foods over high glycemic foods. Consume unrefined extra-virgin olive oil and unrefined virgin coconut oil instead of animal fats and other vegetable oils. The pure unrefined oils supply energy and essential nutrients without causing harm.

As you make changes in your diet, monitor your blood sugar levels regularly. If you are on any medications, take them as prescribed until your doctor tells you they are no longer needed.

3. Eat Regular Meals and Avoid Snacks

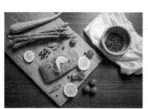
A consistent diet is as important as eating healthy foods. This means eating approximately the same amount of carbohydrates for each meal. You should also eat meals at regular intervals. This helps to avoid blood sugar spikes and evens out your blood sugar levels during the day.

You should not snack unless your blood sugar is low or if the time between meals during the day is greater than five hours. At other times, you should avoid snacks. If you do snack occasionally, choose a low-carb snack without a lot of calories.

It is advisable that you follow a low-carb diet plan of some kind. Your diet is the most important factor you can control to reverse type 2 diabetes and control your blood sugar.

4. Exercise or Walk Daily

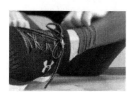

Exercising for 30-60 minutes a day is necessary for naturally controlling diabetes. This kind of physical activity also reduces the chances heart disease, kidney problems and other health complications.

You can select any kind of exercise you like. Brisk walking, jogging, swimming are excellent exercises that increase the heart rate. Choose the exercise that suits you best, and make sure you do it daily. This will help you keep your blood sugar in control and maintain normal cholesterol and triglyceride levels.

5. Control Your Weight and Blood Pressure

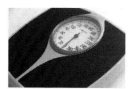

Part of a healthy lifestyle is maintaining proper weight and blood pressure. You should keep up with your blood pressure and weight on a regular basis. Inexpensive weight scales and blood pressure cuffs are available that you can use at home. Your doctor will also monitor these numbers during office visits.

6. Manage Stress and Anxiety

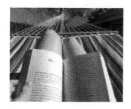

Do not sweat the small stuff–and it is all small stuff anyway. Stop stressing yourself out. Take a walk in the park or walk by the beach. Do whatever it takes to relax your mind and body.

You may need to develop additional problem solving and coping skills to deal with stress and worry. You might talk to your friends or spouse and share your feelings, or you might get some counseling from a qualified counselor, pastor, priest or rabbi. You may also want to try some stress relieving techniques such as breathing exercises.

7. Get a Good Night's Sleep

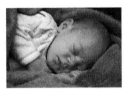
Occasional all-nighters will not have long lasting negative effects, but long-term sleep deprivation is bad for you. Lack of adequate sleep has been linked to chronic diseases such as type 2 diabetes and heart disease. Your body needs time to heal and repair itself during the night. People who sleep seven to eight hours a night eat fewer calories than those who sleep less. Your brain operates better after adequate sleep and your mood improves.

8. Monitor Your Blood Sugar and Lower your A1c

Monitor Your Blood Sugar

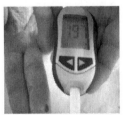
You can easily keep up with own blood sugar levels by self-monitoring them with a device called a glucometer. This random glucose meter test is the method that most people use to self-monitor their blood sugar levels during the day.

Your health care provider can help you devise a monitoring plan. Keeping a record of your blood sugar will help you and your health care provider manage your blood sugar better.

You can buy glucometers at most pharmacies. They are inexpensive to purchase. Pharmacies sometimes have free coupons for glucometers. Then, all you need are the disposable test strips.

Lower Your A1c

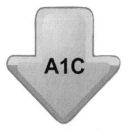

HbA1c, also known as A1c, is a calculation of your average (mean) glucose level over the past three or four months. This lab test helps your doctor understand how you are controlling your blood sugar over time. Glucose meters show your blood sugar level at one point in time and it varies between meals. HbA1c shows your average blood sugar control over a longer period of time.

	HbA1c	Average Blood Glucose Level	
	Test Score	Mg/dl (US)	mmol/L
	14.0	380	21.1
	13.0	350	19.3
Action	12.0	315	17.4
Needed	11.0	280	15.6
	10.0	250	13.7
	9.0	215	11.9
OK	8.0	180	10.0
Good	7.0	150	8.2
	6.0	115	6.3
Excellent	5.0	80	4.7
	4.0	50	2.6

If your HbA1c is below 7, you have done an excellent job of controlling your average blood sugar levels over the past three or four months.

> **The formula for converting HbA1c to common readings in mg/dl is: (HbA1c x 28.7) – 46.8**
>
> If you have an HbA1c reading of 8 then
>
> 8 x 28.7 = 229.6
>
> 229.6-46.8 = 182.8 m

Your HbA1c will go down if control your blood sugar. It will go higher if you do not control your blood sugar. Losing weight and exercising more will help you control your blood sugar levels and lower your HbA1c. Your HbA1c also shows your doctor how well the medicines he has prescribed for you are helping to control your blood sugar.

The Hb in the HbA1c stands for hemoglobin. Hemoglobin is the red protein that transports oxygen in the blood. Glucose likes to attach to the hemoglobin in proteins. Higher blood sugar averages cause more glucose molecules to attach to the hemoglobin. The HbA1c measure this. Red blood cells live approximately 90-120 days. The HbA1c lab test gives you a good view of what your blood sugar levels have been for the past 90-120 days.

You should have an A1c test done routinely during your doctor's visits or you can have it done on your own. See the Additional Resources at the end of the book if you are interested in having this test done yourself without a doctor's order.

9. Lower Your Cholesterol and Triglycerides

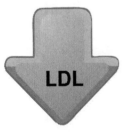

Lab tests can help you monitor the levels of certain lipids (fats) in your blood. These tests show the levels of triglycerides and cholesterol in your blood. These tests should be part of your regular medical exams. Your health care provider can review these lab test results with you and help you understand what they mean for your particular situation.

Tracking all these various numbers from these tests over time will help you see patterns. Your health care provider can also help you set goals with these numbers. You can use these goals to devise an action plan to improve or maintain your numbers. These numbers can be used to measure your progress. You can also review these numbers with someone else for accountability purposes.

10. Stop Smoking and Stop Drinking Alcoholic Beverages

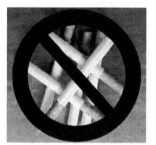

Smoking has absolutely no health benefits. If you have diabetes, you must quit smoking. Yes, it is tough, but you will have to bite the bullet and do it. This is a good decision. It will improve your health and reduce future risks of lung cancer, heart disease and other problems.

Alcohol contains almost twice as many calories as carbs. Alcohol contains seven calories per gram. Carbs contain four calories per gram. Most alcoholic mixed drinks and beer also contain a lot of carbs. Alcohol and alcoholic beverages can cause your blood glucose levels to be unstable. Alcohol tends to increase triglycerides, a type of fat in the blood.

If you have diabetes or prediabetes, do yourself a favor and abstain from alcohol altogether. If you cannot abstain, then make sure you consume it in moderation.

10 Guidelines Recap

People who follow these 10 guidelines will have greater success in managing their blood sugar levels. Adopting these 10 healthy guidelines can also help prevent heart disease, Alzheimer's and dementia. Overall, a healthy eating and exercise routine can add years to your life and reduce your risk from the disabling complications of diabetes and other diseases.

Here is a recap of these 10 guidelines:

---

10 Guidelines for Type 2 Diabetes Blood Sugar Management

1. Avoid unhealthy carbohydrates and fats
2. Select the right foods in the right amounts
3. Eat regular meals and avoid snacks
4. Exercise or walk daily
5. Control your weight and blood pressure
6. Manage stress and anxiety
7. Get a good night's sleep
8. Control your blood sugar and lower your A1c
9. Lower your blood cholesterol and triglycerides
10. Stop smoking and stop drinking alcoholic beverages

These 10 guidelines reflect an overall healthy living perspective that forms the foundation for controlling the symptoms of type 2 diabetes and prediabetes. They focus more on blood sugar management for type 2 diabetes more than anything else.

These guidelines are not meant to be a comprehensive list for diabetic care. Your health care provider will advise you and provide recommendations for your particular situation. You may need more exams to ensure your eyes, kidneys and feet are healthy. You may also need specialized care for diabetic complications.

For most people, those without serious complications, this list can serve as a starting point to manage and lower high blood sugar levels on a day-to-day basis. It is important to understand that additional steps and actions are necessary for most type 2 diabetes to be reversed and enter into remission.

Summary of Type 2 Diabetes Reversal Solutions

In this part of the book, we have discovered how diabetes reversal is possible. Weight-loss surgery and very low-calorie, low-carb diets have been successful in reversing type 2 diabetes. After weight-loss surgery, type 2 diabetes reversal can occur in a few days. With very low-calorie, low-carb diets, results can take approximately eight weeks or longer.

Type 2 diabetes is linked to obesity, but weight-loss surgery demonstrates that diabetes can be reversed without significant initial weight loss. Weight-loss surgery is not ideal for reversing diabetes because of its complications and additional risks associated with removing parts of the stomach and digestive system.

Very low-calorie, low-carb diets were studied by Dr. Roy Taylor at Newcastle University in the UK. This most is the most promising study that demonstrated type 2 diabetes could be reversed in eight weeks using a very low-calorie, low-carb diet.

Not all patients in the Newcastle study were successful in reversing their diabetes. Before participants started the study, they were checked to see how much insulin their pancreases were secreting. Their pancreases' ability to produce insulin predicted whether the very low-calorie, low-carb diet would be successful or not.

After a few years, some who have type 2 diabetes may have their pancreas beta cells stop producing adequate amounts of insulin to maintain proper blood sugar levels. Then they must take insulin. This seems to be a factor in whether type 2 diabetes can be reversed or not.

At the end of the study, participants who had type 2 diabetes longer than 10 years and did not produce insulin normally, were not successful at reversing their diabetes. However, they were successful in losing weight and gaining better control over their blood sugar levels. The program did provide some worthwhile results for them.

Some participants in the Newcastle study who were taking insulin and had been diagnosed for fewer than 10 years were able to see their type 2 diabetes reverse or go into remission. This effect continued after the eight-week program was over and the remission was still intact six months later.

This is very good news for those who are newly diagnosed with type 2 diabetes and for those who have had type 2 diabetes for less than 10 years. They have the possibility of seeing their type 2 diabetes reverse so they no longer have to take drugs or insulin.

It has been noted that the sudden restriction on the amount of food eaten causes the fat inside the pancreas and the liver to be reduced dramatically. This occurs right after weight-loss surgery or while on a very low-calorie, low-carb diet. This may be the reason their pancreases can produce more insulin. It may also help explain why insulin sensitivity is also regained.

When insulin production increases and insulin sensitivity is regained, blood sugar levels return to normal. Exercise also increases insulin sensitivity, but a very low-calorie, low-carb diet can completely reverse type 2 diabetes in many cases.

Here is a link to an MRI of a study participant's liver before and after they finished the eight-week New Castle very low-calorie, low-carb diet study.

https://www.diabetes.org.uk/Global/Research/DiRECT%20-%20MRI%20scan.jpg

Notice there is a significant reduction in the amount of fat visible inside the liver after the completion of the eight-week very low-calorie, low-carb diet. The diet produced a sharp decrease in the amount of fat in this liver from 36% to 2%.

The article explaining these results can be found at:

https://www.diabetes.org.uk/Research/Research-round-up/Research-spotlight/Research-spotlight-low-calorie-liquid-diet/

There are some other links to the Newcastle study listed earlier in this step in the section about how low-calorie, low-carb diets can reverse type 2 diabetes.

A very low-calorie, low-carb diet program can be a great way to jumpstart your lifestyle changes and lose weight rapidly. It is recommended that you continue to follow the guidelines and exercise or walk for at least 30 minutes a day or more if possible. This will ensure that the benefits of this weight loss are sustainable.

Once you control your blood sugar levels or reverse your diabetes, you want to keep the progress you have made. This can be achieved with permanent changes in eating and exercise habits. Again, the guidelines to manage your blood sugar listed above will help you tremendously if you follow them and put them into action.

A very low-calorie, low-carb diet can be incorporated into a complete plan to help you reverse or control your type 2 diabetes. The next step in this book, Step 3, will show you how to create such a plan. This plan will build upon the principles and guidelines outlined in this part of the book, Step 2.

The last step in the book, Step 4, will briefly review action plans that that others are already using that includes knowledge about low-calorie, low-carb diets, fasting, nutrition, exercise and weight loss.

The Additional Resources section at the very end of the book provides links to the action plans mentioned in Step 4. There are also links to more information and action plans that could be useful for diabetes reversal and management.

Reversal of type 2 diabetes is possible for most people. However, action and commitment are required to accomplish this goal. The journey to get there is not so easy for most people. It is difficult to for most people to change a lifetime of eating habits and sedentary living. It is possible to change for the better, and many people have undertaken this journey and have successfully completed it.

This book has presented the facts and principles of weight loss and type 2 diabetes reversal. Now, take the next step on your journey. Develop an action plan and stick to it.

> *A very low-calorie, low-carb diet is not something that is easy to do for eight weeks. However, this is the solution to reverse type 2 diabetes for most people. The initial effort to follow an action plan like this for eight weeks can pay a lifetime of dividends to you.*

Even if you stumble on your journey, keep the benefits of the goal in front of you. Imagine your life free from the effects of type 2 diabetes. See yourself accomplishing this goal. Be determined to accomplish it. Put forth the effort, have courage and develop the self-control needed. Start taking daily steps toward your goal, and you will succeed in living a healthier life, and in many cases, completely reverse your type 2 diabetes.

The information in this book will help even those who cannot reverse their diabetes to prevent additional complications that could be caused by high blood sugar. The information in this book when put into action is useful for all types of situations whether diabetes is reversed completely or not.

Even if you do not choose to undertake an eight-week very low-calorie, low-carb diet, you still need to develop and follow some kind of action plan to manage and control your blood sugar levels. A good plan when followed can help avoid severe complications caused by out-of-control blood sugar.

Step 3: Develop an Action Plan to Reverse Diabetes

The Importance of Having Goals and Plans

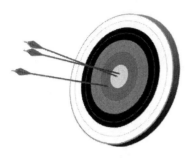

There is a saying by the late Zig Ziglar,

If you aim at nothing, you will hit it every time."

Benjamin Franklin, one of the founding fathers of the United States said,

If you fail to plan, you are planning to fail.

Another popular saying that has been around for at least 200 years is:

Plan your work and work your plan.

Failing to plan most often leads to failure. Not following through with hard work and effort in achieving your plan will also lead to failure. You have to be motivated to plan and follow the plan before you will accomplish the plan.

Unfortunately, few people plan and even fewer people write their goals down. People with clear written goals accomplish far more than most people without them. Written goals will help you measure your progress towards success. They act as targets to focus your valuable time and energy. This helps you overcome obstacles and keep moving forward. Written goals can also provide accountability. The process of making and writing down goals is a powerful motivation tool that helps you to achieve real results in the real world.

Every football team or soccer team has a goal to win a championship of some kind. Every team develops a game plan to help them reach their goal of winning a championship. Because they have a game plan, they do not wander up and down the field aimlessly.

They use their game plan to overcome their opponents and score points. They work hard to follow their game plan. They practice, drill and rehearse their plans before they are ready to enter the playing field. Then on game day, they do their best to follow their game plan. Their game plan helps them play one play at a time and win one game at a time.

A team without a good game plan will not win many games or a championship no matter how talented they are. Some of the best players are on teams that never win championships. A good game plan is necessary for a team to win games and a championship. A good game plan helps the team to play to their fullest potential.

Apollo 13 moon mission commander, James Lovell, said,

> *There are people who make things happen, there are people who watch things happen, and there are people who wonder what happened. To be successful, you need to be a person who makes things happen.*

Planning is important for sports teams winning a championship, starting a space colony on Mars or managing a business. Planning is important for you to bring about changes in your life. Goals and plans help you to take aim at the bullseye of the target. They help guide you towards success.

Anything worth accomplishing is worth the time and effort to think through the options and develop a written plan for success. Goals that are written are no longer vague ideas or random thoughts. They become tangible words that allow you to become accountable to yourself and others. Goals and plans help you manage time, money and energy. If circumstance change, goals enable you to change directions when adjustments need to be made to correct your course of action.

Goals provide a timeline to determine how well you are doing. Written goals will help you when you get bogged down and need to focus on accomplishing something. Goals help you to see your weaknesses and develop further actions to overcome them. Once goals are achieved, they bring great satisfaction and bring with them the rewards of success.

People with clear written goals accomplish far more than most people without them. Writing down your goals and developing a good plan of action separates you from the multitudes with good intentions, wishful thinking and unclear pathways to success.

SMART Goals

A successful plan should have written goals that are Specific, Measurable, Accountable, Realistic and Timely. The Acronym SMART will help you remember the basics of successful goal setting.

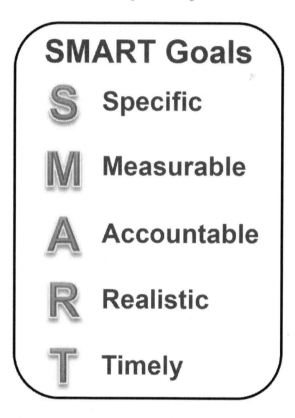

SMART Goals

S Specific

M Measurable

A Accountable

R Realistic

T Timely

Specific. Specific goals are clearly defined. Who will take action and what will they do? A goal creates a definite statement of intention. Having a goal to lose weight is not specific. Having a goal to lose 25 pounds by a certain date pounds is more specific. Having a goal to lower your blood sugar is not specific. Having a goal to lower your HBa1C average blood sugar to below 7 in six months is a specific goal.

Measurable. You should be able to have some concrete measurement of how much or how many. If your goal is not measurable, how will you know if you achieved it? What are the units of measurement that you will use to set your goals? Successful goals have measurable results. Mile signs on the highway help you see how far you have come and how far you need to go to reach your destination.

Accountable. Goals often fail because of a lack of accountability. When other people are involved in some way, this motivates you to achieve your goals. Accountability makes you responsible for your actions. Having someone to be accountable to raises your level of commitment to achieve your goals. Accountability is more obvious in a team or business environment. Accountability for individual goals can be trickier. Recruiting a friend or family member to hold you accountable will help you ensure success for your personal goals.

Realistic. Do not set goals so high that they are not obtainable. Losing 10 pounds overnight is not realistic or achievable. Goals should be realistic enough to be challenging and require some effort to accomplish. Do not set goals so low that they are too easy to meet.

Timely. Goals need a completion date. Set a time frame to finish the goal. This helps you have a sense of urgency. Set a date and avoid doing everything at the last minute. Set up steps and timelines within the goal to accomplish certain measurable results. Goals can have short-term or long-term timelines.

SMART Goals Are More than Resolutions

Look at a typical New Year's resolution "I am going to lose weight starting on January 1." Losing weight is a great aim, but by itself is not a SMART goal. There is no Specific, Measurable, Accountable and Timely aspect to it. The only thing this goal has going for it is that it is realistic. People do lose weight all the time, but to be a SMART goal it needs to have **S**pecific, **M**easurable, **A**ccountable, **R**ealistic and **T**imely components combined.

Revise the goal, "I am going to lose weight starting on January 1." to, "I am going to lose 25 pounds in six months starting on January, 1, and I will be accountable to my personal trainer." This is a smart goal because it is **S**pecific, **M**easurable, **A**ccountable, **R**ealistic and **T**imely.

Strategies or Methods

A goal is a statement of the desired result. Strategies are the broad methods that are utilized to achieve the goal. The goal serves as the specific desired result while the strategy defines the system, program or means used to accomplish the goal.

Suppose your goal is to lose 25 pounds in 6 months. What are your strategies to accomplish this goal? How will you go about this? Will you exercise, change your diet or have weight-loss surgery? These are all strategies or methods. Let us eliminate weight-loss surgery as too risky an option. This leaves you with many diet and exercise strategy options.

You can combine several exercise and diet strategies. For exercise, you can walk in the park, ride a bike, swim or weight train. Diet changes can be accomplished by finding one of many diet programs that fit your lifestyle, personal tastes and preferences.

Tactics or Action Steps

Once you have decided upon the broad strategies you will use to accomplish your goals, your focus will shift to developing action steps associated with your strategies. Action steps are necessary to carry out the strategies you chose to achieve your goals. Your action steps are the specific tactics you will use to accomplish your goals and strategies. Your action steps state how you will utilize your energy, time and money to accomplish your goals and strategies. Your actions steps along with your goals and strategies create a workable plan.

Action Steps for accomplishing your weight loss goals and strategy could be to obtain a gym membership and enroll in an aerobics class three times a week and weight train two days a week. Alternatively, you could buy a mountain bike and ride 5 hours a week. You could use any combination of exercises such as running, dancing, swimming or whatever you prefer.

You might choose the Diabetes Destroyer program strategy. Your Phase 1 action steps for this diet might be to buy a blender. Then you would shop for the ingredients for the smoothies, fresh vegetable soups and salads for the first 10 days. Then you would have action steps for Phase 2 of the action plan for the next 8 weeks.

A Simple Action Plan to Lose 25 Pounds

Planning can be simple or complex. The simplest form of planning involves setting goals, developing strategies and developing a plan of action to accomplish those goals and strategies.

A fully functional plan will include goals, strategies and action steps.

Goal: I will lose 25 pounds in the next six months, and I will share my progress and be accountable to my spouse.

Exercise Strategy: I will lose weight by a combination of walking and weight training.

Exercise Action Steps

- I will buy a good pair of running shoes today.
- I will join a gym near my house
- I will buy and use a fitness tracker watch.
- I will walk one hour a day five times a week in the park.
- I will weight train in the gym two times a week.
- I will find an accountability buddy in the gym.
- I will measure my weight three times a week.
- I will share my weight measurements with my spouse.

Diet Strategy: I will follow a low-calorie, low-carbohydrate diet and limit my calorie intake to 1000 calories a day. I will also have one day a week to eat 2000 calories. I will be accountable to my best friend.

Diet Action Steps

- I will keep a meal and snack log and calculate my daily calorie intake from it.
- I will research and buy a diet plan product that fits my tastes.
- I will clean out my refrigerator and pantry and remove unhealthy foods and drinks
- I will stop drinking soft drinks and sugary snacks.
- I will shop for only healthy foods and eliminate all processed foods and starchy snacks.
- I will only use healthy oils like extra-virgin olive oil or coconut oil.
- I will follow the 1,000-calorie diet plan 6 days a week on Sunday I will eat 2,000 calories.
- I will meet with my best friend and discuss my results weekly.

Plan Your Work–Speak Your Plan–Work Your Plan

What did I say? I said, "Plan your work–speak your plan–work your plan." I added the phrase speak your plan to the phrase "plan your work–work your plan. Why did I do this? It may sound crazy to some people, but successful people say what they are planning to do before they do it.

When you hear yourself say what you are going to do, it builds faith inside you to accomplish something positive. People often speak their worries out loud. They convince themselves that what they are worrying about will come to pass. They create a negative atmosphere with their own words. Why not do the opposite. Instead of speaking your worries, speak out your SMART goals, strategies and action lists. Create a positive atmosphere with positive statements.

When you speak your plan, you will create an image of success in your mind. This image helps motivate you towards your goal. This image keeps you going when times get tough and things look like they are not working.

Notice how the following goal, strategy and action steps are easy to say out loud. As you speak you goal strategy and action steps, you will see yourself completing them in six months. You can also imagine what you will look like and feel like when you are 25 pounds lighter.

Goal: I will lose 25 pounds in the next six months, and I will share my progress with my accountability buddy.

Exercise Strategy: I will lose weight by a combination of walking and weight training.

Exercise Action Steps

- I will walk one hour a day five times a week in the park.
- I will weight train in the gym two times a week.
- I will find an accountability buddy in the gym.

Reading this exercise plan out loud will help you envision its accomplishment. Speaking out the plan will also motivate you to take the action steps to accomplish the plan. If you speak this plan out loud to someone you want to be accountable to, it will add further motivation to complete it. It might also be helpful to set up a reward for yourself that you can share with your accountability buddy when you accomplish your plan and achieve the weight loss.

Additional Considerations When Developing Goals and Plans

Successful goal setting is part of an overall understanding of the many facets of your life. Your plans and goals should reflect who you are and what you have experienced. Goals and plans are statements of future expectations, but they are built on the reality of who you are now. Who you want to become in the future is affected by who you are now and the circumstances of life.

What is Your Purpose in Life?

The foundation for a great plan is built upon a great purpose or mission for your life. Why do you want to be healthy? Who do you want to be healthy for? It helps to have meaning or a sense of mission in your life before you set out to set specific goals.

Your goals can change your current circumstances and create a new life for you, but you do not want to just dream up goals out of a vacuum. If you take a little time to examine your life before you set your goals, you will be more successful in the long run.

Understanding your purpose or mission in life is not always obvious. What kind of person do you want to be? What are your core values? What principles do you wish to follow in your life? Who is important to you?

Here are some things you might write down when examining your purpose. These may help you discover your values and help you understand why you want to be healthy.

- What would motivate you to excellence?
- What past successes are important to you?
- What contributions do you want to make to those around you?

Once you finish your soul searching for your most important values, you might even write a brief mission statement for yourself before you start setting goals.

What Are Your Strengths, Weaknesses, Opportunities and Challenges?

What are your talents, strengths and limitations? Understanding your situation and current circumstances are also important background information for creating realistic and specific goals. Exercise plans, in particular, are affected by physical limitations. Choose your goals to fit well within your combination of talents, strengths and weaknesses.

What are the opportunities and challenges that will have the greatest impact on your life? These could be things from your past or things that loom in the future. Your goals should reflect the opportunities and challenges in your life that will affect your decisions for the future.

Make a Few Assumptions before Planning

Certain assumptions should also be made before you make your plans. These should involve your circumstances now and how they might change or remain the same in the future. If you are moving, graduating or changing careers, this could affect your plans. Make assumptions about these future changes and adjust your plans accordingly.

Your plans might include some other broad assumptions such as:

- Your goals and plans should be good for you. They should not do more harm than good to you and others.
- You are willing and able to apply the time and effort necessary to achieve your goals and plans.
- Goals and plans should be positively stated. Negativity should not be included.

Good planning should be based upon your purpose in life and other factors that affect our ability to carry out your goals. Once you look at other factors such as your talents, strengths and weaknesses, you are well on your way to creating goals that fit well with your life. You should develop goals that take advantage of your opportunities and minimize the challenges in your life.

Allow for Some Flexibility in Your Plans

Plans should not be written in stone. Your plans should be realistic plans that have achievable, realistic goals. You should set certain dates during the progress of your plan to review your goals. If needed, at these review dates, you can revise your plan rather than completely abandoning it.

Plans need some flexibility because circumstances sometimes change quickly. Perhaps, the plan needs changing because the goals were not realistic in the first place. Maybe, you did a good job setting your goal, but your strategy to carry out the goal may not have been the right one.

If your strategy to lose weight involved swimming and this did not work out. Maybe, it was because you had to make frequent trips to a pool that was not near your home. In this case, you might find a pool closer to your home, or you could change your strategy to walking or something else that you can do at nearby park or beach.

Do not give up the goal because of a strategy that did not work as you expected it to work. You might have to try different types of strategies to find out what works best for you. You might also get bored with the same strategy. Then, you should not give up your goal. You should find a more interesting or challenging strategy to carry out your goals

Suppose your goal and strategy were right for you, but your tactics to carry out the goals and strategies were not working. Your tactics in your action plan may have called for three days of walking followed by 2 days of weight lifting. Maybe you could change your tactics to walking 2 days a week and weight lifting 3 days a week. Alternatively, you might substitute a bike ride on the weekend for one the days of walking.

Do not throw out plans if your goals, strategies and tactics are not working. Revise and modify your plan as needed to reach your goals.

Review Your Plan upon Completion

After you fulfill your timeline for your goals, you should do a complete review of the entire plan including all your goals, strategies and tactics. This kind of feedback is valuable information that will help you when you make future plans.

You will want to continue to have a plan for your health and fitness for the rest of your life. What worked well? What did not work at all? What might have worked better if you had made some changes?

You should view planning as an ongoing operation. Once you go through the cycle of creating goals, strategies and action lists and revising them a few times, you will get better at the skill of planning. You will continue to see yourself spending your time wisely and taking realistic, measurable actions to accomplish more and more worthwhile goals.

Reward Yourself for Achieving Your Goal

During challenging times, it helps when you consider the rewards of success rather than worrying about the problems. A positive attitude is necessary for achieving success. Thinking about your rewards will help you stick to your goals when your will is weak or you are facing adverse circumstances. Have faith and confidence in what you are doing. Your future rewards help you to believe your goal is worth the time, effort and determination needed to achieve it.

Do not become negative. Think about the rewards you will give yourself once you achieve your goals. If your goal was to lose weight, plan to reward yourself when with some new clothes in a smaller size.

Make your rewards fun. Plan to buy something or do something you always wanted to do. Plan to take a trip or vacation. Plan a celebration to share what you have accomplished with your friends and family. This might encourage some of them to follow in your footsteps. Think about how your success will be an inspiration for them to lead healthier lives.

A Complete Plan Includes SMART Goals, Strategies and Action Steps

Having a SMART goal is not the same as having a complete plan. Plans must also include strategies and have action items that will be followed. In real life, people may have only pieces of a plan. These pieces can provide some benefit, but it is not likely they will result in any substantial success.

Strategies without Goals. Going to the gym or adopting a certain kind of diet is a strategy. You can gain some benefit from going to the gym, but without a goal, how will you know you are finished with your strategy? Strategies work best when they are coupled with a goal that is **S**pecific, **M**easurable, **A**ccountable and **T**imely.

Goals without Strategies. The goals may be **S**pecific, **M**easurable, **A**ccountable, **R**ealistic and **T**imely but it will never get off the ground without a strategy. You must choose a method to accomplish your goal. What exercise program will you use to accomplish your goal? What diet program will you adopt to lose weight? A goal must have a strategy to move forward.

Goals and Strategies without Action Lists. If you have a SMART goal and a strategy that does not include actionable items to go with the strategies, you still do not have a plan. You just have an exercise in wishful thinking.

A complete plan will have a SMART goal, a well thought out strategy and detailed action steps. If you have all three of these present, you have a functional plan. A simple plan with these three parts is much more powerful than just pieces of the plan by themselves.

Goal: I will bring my A1c below 7 in 6 months and be accountable to my spouse.

Strategy1: I will use the Diabetes Destroyer 8-week nutrition program.

Action Steps. **1.** I will walk shop for the necessary food Items. **2.** I will choose one meal plan for breakfast ... **3** ... **4** ... **5** ... etc.

Suggested Areas for Smart Goals and Plans

SMART goal planning should be done for all of the areas that are important for managing and reversing type 2 diabetes. You can use any of these suggested areas that follow to develop detailed personalized goals, strategies and action lists to accomplish them. They reflect the general guidelines I have recommended earlier to reverse type 2 diabetes.

A Few Suggested Areas
For Goal Setting and Planning

- Controlling the types and amounts of food eaten
- Eliminating unhealthy fats and carbohydrates.
- Maintaining consistent eating patterns and habits.
- Regular exercise.
- Reducing stress and anxiety.
- Getting help for addictions to drugs, alcohol or tobacco.
- Reducing blood pressure, weight and lipid profile numbers.
- Managing your diabetes medicines and appointments.
- Reducing or eliminating your diabetes medicines.
  (Planned together with your healthcare team or physician)
- Receiving care for diabetic complications.

SMART Goal Confidence Ladder

How confident are you in accomplishing your goals? Your level of confidence will determine your level of success in reaching your goal.

Where are you on the confidence ladder? Have you convinced yourself that there is a certainty to the accomplishment of your SMART goals?

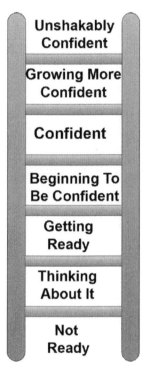

Not Ready. At the bottom of the confidence ladder, you are standing there wondering if you can accomplish your goal. You are not ready to start working towards your goal just yet.

Thinking about It. You begin to think about your goal more and more and this takes you to the next step on the confidence ladder.

Getting Ready. At this step, you go about getting ready to take action on your goal, and you begin to be confident about what you are going to do. You establish a **SMART** goal, a goal that is, **S**pecific, **M**easurable, **A**ccountable, **R**ealistic and **T**imely.

Confident. You take your SMART goal, develop a strategy and action steps. You have a functional action plan. Then, you begin taking actions and you are confident your SMART goal is achievable.

Growing in Confidence. You have set your goals, and you have made strategies and started taking actions steps towards your goal. You grow in confidence as you begin to measure your progress. You continue to measure your progress, and you grow in confidence with each action step.

Unshakably Confident. You believe you will be successful. You have reached the point of no return. You are accountable to someone and your progress continues to move forward. Your confidence has grown to the point it is unshakeable. You are convinced you will receive the benefits of your goal and experience the rewards of your success.

If you never plan, you are planning to fail. So, do not plan to fail. Just do it. Take the time to make a plan with SMART goals, strategies and action steps. Then take action. You will grow in confidence with each step until you have an unshakeable confidence that you will reach your goal.

You may not feel confident at first and this is expected. Keep going through the process, and you will grow in confidence, and then your actions will achieve the results you want. Boldly declare your plan and then follow it to the end. You may find yourself pleasantly surprised at how well the process works.

The Difference between Confidence and Overconfidence

Here are a few more thoughts about confidence. There is a difference between genuine confidence and overconfidence. Overconfidence is a form of arrogance and entitlement. Overconfidence arises from a lack of humility and an unrealistic assessment of your abilities to accomplish or complete a task.

If you have taken the time to develop genuine confidence in your goals and plans, you will accomplish them. If you believe you should accomplish your plans without work or effort on your part, you are deceiving yourself, and you might be suffering from the negative forces of overconfidence. This type of overconfidence is a barrier to your success.

If you keep an honest and realistic assessment of yourself and your goals, your confidence will become reality based and unshakeable. This genuine confidence will empower you to achieve great things.

Even if you do not feel like you are confident if you believe your plans will work, boldly take the first step, and then the next. If you have a good plan, your action steps will lead you to success.

True confidence is not based upon some emotion are feeling of self-importance. True confidence is based on being fully persuaded you will accomplish your worthwhile goals and action steps.

Slaying the Giant and Defeating Diabetes

In the Bible, there is a story about a teenage shepherd named David. This young man had the confidence to go out and slay a giant with a sling and a stone. You can find this story in the Old Testament part of the Bible in the book of 1 Samuel and Chapter 17.

In the story, there was a giant named Goliath who was 9 feet tall. He wore heavy armor. He had a spear that was over 20 feet long (6 m), and the spear tip weighed 18 pounds (8 kg). He was a veteran warrior. Every day he would go out and challenge the opposing army where David's brothers were soldiers. One day David came to bring food to his brothers. They were all afraid to go out and fight against the giant.

David knew the king was going to give great rewards to anyone who would slay the giant. David had already killed a lion and a bear that had attacked his father's flock of sheep. David had the faith and confidence that he could also defeat the giant. He knew God was on his side. He had experience, and he had a plan, a strategy and a detailed action plan.

David's King was impressed with David. He agreed to let him fight the giant. He even offered him his own armor and weapons, but David refused them. David's strategy was to use what was familiar to him. He was going to use his sling and stones. His action plan was to strike down the giant with his sling and stones. Then, he was going to cut off his head.

David boldly declared his goal. He told the giant he was going to kill him and cut off his head. He told the giant that the whole world would know God was on his side. He went on to battle the heavily armored giant who was mocking him and cursing him because of his small size. He knocked the giant down by hitting him right between the eyes with one of the stones from the sling. Then, he ran toward the giant and cut the giant's head off with the giant's own sword. He overcame the giant that day in battle, and he became a great hero to his countrymen.

David had a plan. He had a strategy. He took action. He accomplished his goal. He received the king's rewards and was given the king's daughter as his wife. The whole world became aware that God was on his side that day. He went on later to become a great king, and people all over the world still talk about the story of David killing Goliath 3,000 years later.

The moral of the story is that David saw a problem. He was confident that with God's help he could slay the giant. He had a plan. He had the right strategy and equipment. He declared his intentions to the giant and everyone listening. He then set out and took bold action steps. He achieved his goal and killed the giant, and then, he received the rewards and satisfaction of his achievement.

You can use the same concepts David used to overcome the giant of diabetes in your life that is cursing you and threatening to kill you. You can set your goal, choose your strategy and take decisive action. You can develop the faith and confidence to achieve victory over diabetes. You can inspire others and give them something to talk about. You can overcome diabetes and celebrate victory over your enemy!

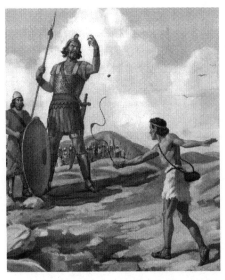

David and Goliath Painting by Robert Ayres
License CC By 2.0

Step 4: Implement an Action Plan to Reverse Diabetes

No plan is complete without the implementation of strategies with action steps. Strategies are the methods by which the goals can be accomplished. Diet plans and exercise plans are strategies that can be used to accomplish weight loss goals and blood sugar control goals. Strategies then need be broken down into detailed action plans. The following diet and exercise plans can be used to implement detailed action plans to help you achieve your SMART goals to lose weight, control your blood sugar levels or to possibly reverse type 2 diabetes.

Walking

One of the simplest and most effective exercise strategies around to lose weight and control your blood sugar is walking. Best of all, this strategy is free. You might need a new pair of walking shoes, but other than that, you can implement this strategy without spending a dime.

Almost everyone can implement a walking strategy to accomplish his or her goals. Unless you have some physical limitations where you cannot walk, you should develop a goal that has a walking strategy with a detailed action plan.

It is not just enough to have a goal to walk more every day. You should have a SMART goal to walk more. As we have already mentioned a **SMART** goal is **S**pecific, **M**easurable, **A**ccountable, **R**ealistic and **T**imely.

The American Diabetes Association has a great page with tips about walking. You can find it here:

http://www.diabetes.org/food-and-fitness/fitness/types-of-activity/walking-a-great-place-to-start.html

On this page, you can download a detailed starter-walking plan.

http://main.diabetes.org/dorg/PDFs/walking-plan.pdf

Except for accountability, this 12-week action plan includes all the elements to help you reach a SMART exercise goal. Accountability can be added by sharing your plan with someone else. This person will agree to hold you accountable for taking action steps and reaching your goals.

If you own a smartphone, it is easy to measure your daily steps in your action plan. You can find apps that will do this for you. You can set the app to count your steps automatically in the background.

Noom, Inc. has free pedometer app, Noom Walk Pedometer. This a good app with some nice features. It can be integrated with another Noom app, Noom Coach. Together, they will keep up with your daily steps and calories for each meal. The coaching app provides coaching advice, tracks your weight and helps you set goals for your daily calorie limits. You can download both of these free apps from the Apple Store (iTunes) or the Google Play Store. The Noom Coach also has an upgraded version with more features. A link for this with more information is included in the Additional Resources section at the end of the book.

If you do not own a smartphone, you can keep track of your daily steps with an inexpensive pedometer. You can find these as sports stores and other retailers. The little device clicks on to your belt or clothes. This device gives you an ongoing total of your daily steps.

Everyone should have a SMART exercise goal and strategy to walk so many steps a day. If you are out of shape, you can start slow with less than 1,000 steps a day and build up to 5,000 or 6,000 steps a day. If you are in good shape, you might set your goal to 10,000 steps a day.

Your walking strategy can be implemented along with other diet and exercise strategies and plans.

The Newcastle University Research Diet

If you are diabetic, you should be supervised or receive the advice of your health care provider before trying to duplicate any research using low-calorie, low-carb diets on your own. Your medicine dosages may need adjustments to avoid low blood sugar problems. None of this information should be considered as a substitute for medical advice for your individual situation.

The most successful type 2 diabetes reversal diet was developed at Newcastle University in the UK. Dr. Rod Taylor led the original research study. He designed the research diet to resemble the prescribed diet for a person who had undergone stomach bypass surgery (bariatric surgery).

Stomach bypass surgery has been known for 20 years to cause diabetes reversal. This study proved it is possible to reverse type 2 diabetes by following the bariatric surgery diet without having the surgery and its dangerous side effects.

When the diet from the research study was strictly followed, the results were significant. Diabetes reversal means patients were able to stop taking medicines for diabetes. Six months later, they were still not taking medicines to control the symptoms of type 2 diabetes.

The research found the diet could reverse type 2 diabetes in cases where the participants had diabetes for less than 10 years. For those who had type 2 diabetes for 10 years or longer, the diet provided greater blood sugar control, but it did not completely reverse the disease.

If you are lucky enough to live near Newcastle University in the UK where studies to reverse type 2 diabetes are still being conducted, you might volunteer for this program, but for most people, this is not possible.

However, there are some things we can learn from this research that can be used to create type 2 diabetes reversal strategies. Keep in mind that these are physician-monitored programs.

Some key points to remember concerning the original successful research by Dr. Rod Taylor at New Castle University are:

- The study lasted 8 weeks
- The diet consisted of a total of 800 calories a day
- There were three liquid protein based drinks daily (600 calories))
- There were three portions of non-starchy vegetable salads or soups per day (200 calories)
- Everyone was required to drink 2 to 3 liters a day of water or calorie-free fluids
- The diet eliminated dairy products, all meat, pulses (beans, peas), fruits, breads and pastas.
- Alcoholic drinks were not permitted.

If you try to follow a diet similar to this, you may find it desirable to modify these points to fit your lifestyle and needs. You may need to adjust your calorie intake upwards to take into consideration your current health situation. You could also include along with this diet strategy some kind of exercise strategy.

Before you begin this strict kind of diet, or one similar to it, you might want to start a transition diet. This is where you cut back on the amount of food you eat, and you start eliminating dairy products and meat for a couple of weeks before you begin the strict very low-calorie, low-carb diet.

Here is an Internet link to Newcastle University's public information page for diabetes reversal:

http://www.ncl.ac.uk/magres/research/diabetes/reversal/#publicinformation

Here is a link from the above page where you can read a pdf leaflet with information about how their research was conducted:

http://www.ncl.ac.uk/media/wwwnclacuk/newcastlemagneticresonancece ntre/files/reversing-type2-diabetes-leaflet.pdf

The Diabetes Destroyer Program

David Andrews has created a diabetes reversal program that has been successful. This program is named "Diabetes Destroyer." This program follows a similar plan to the one originally developed for the Newcastle Diabetes Reversal Study. The Diabetes Destroyer program is not an exact duplication of the Newcastle diet, but it follows similar principles. The results have proven positive for producing type 2 diabetes reversals in many people. The trick is to strictly follow the eight-week program.

Phase 1 of the Diabetes Destroyer program includes a protein shake type of diet that also includes non-starchy vegetables for the first ten days. The total calories a day is little more than 1,000. Phase 2 substitutes a few more low-carb meal choices for some of the shakes. Vegetables are also an important part of Phase 1 and 2. They keep you filled up and provide needed digestive fiber.

The Diabetes Destroyer program can be used as a strategy to implement your diabetes reversal goal. This program also includes some simple exercises to help you burn more calories. It would also work well with a daily walking exercise strategy or with other exercise strategies such as the Diabetes 60 System.

Thousands of people have already purchased the Diabetes Destroyer program, and many who have stuck with it, have obtained their goal of reversing prediabetes or type 2 diabetes. This means their A1c and blood sugar levels returned to normal.

It is important to understand that these programs will not work without applying effort to understand what is required. They will require your time to follow the actions steps. The Diabetes Destroyer program will require you to buy the necessary food items necessary to follow the action steps. You may also have to purchase a blender.

The Diabetes Destroyer program and other health-related programs are essentially strategies with action plans. Before using any of them, you should develop your own goals and set up the completion dates for yourself. Once you add your measurable and accountable aspects to the strategies and action steps in the Diabetes Destroyer program, and other diet and exercise programs, it will make them into complete plans.

Most of these programs, including the Diabetes Destroyer program, have been designed by people who have already obtained the goals you want to achieve. This means they have already blazed a trail for you to follow. You do not have to reinvent the wheel or try some hit or miss approach. You can follow their advice on what really works based on their real-life experiences. Their strategies and action steps are there for you to adapt and use to accomplish your specific goals. If needed, you can also make changes in their action steps to better fit your situation and circumstances.

Following a well-developed strategy with detailed action steps will help you reach your goals more quickly than trying to come up with a diabetes reversal solution on your own. Following in other's footsteps will keep you from wasting your valuable time and energy. When you follow their already prepared plans, you can focus your time and effort towards reaching your goals. This will keep you from a hit or miss approach from starting from scratch.

Please excuse this high glycemic, sugary analogy, but it explains my point. If grandma makes great apple pies, you might want to follow her recipe for success if you want to bake a pie like hers. You might try to make one from experimenting with the ingredients until you get something close, but it would be much easier and save you time if you followed her recipe. The Diabetes Destroyer is a proven recipe for success.

For readers of this book who purchase the Diabetes Destroyer program the author of this book is offering a free bonus. The bonus is a detailed action plan to get you off to a fast start. It highlights the most important parts of the program and shows you were to begin. See the Action Plan Discounts and Bonuses page at the back of the book for more details.

Fasting and Intermittent Fasting

Historically, insulin was discovered in 1921. Soon after its discovery, doctors figured out how to treat the symptoms of diabetes with insulin. The discovery of insulin has been one of the most important discoveries in medicine. Before the discovery of insulin, the only treatment for diabetes was fasting. The progression of diabetes could be slowed down with fasting, but diabetes was usually a death sentence. Once insulin was discovered, the attention was turned away from fasting to treatment with insulin and other medicines. The difference between type 1 and type 2 diabetes was not understood at this time. They successfully treated type 1 diabetes with insulin. The rise in type 2 diabetes is a more recent phenomenon.

The increase of stomach bypass surgeries in the past 20 years has proven that there is a link between the surgery and the remission of type 2 diabetes. A significant number of patients with type 2 diabetes had their diabetes go into complete remission shortly after the surgery. The remission of the disease was not linked to the amount of weight they lost. Many patients who had little or no weight loss saw their diabetes symptoms go into remission.

Weight-loss surgery is a type of forced fasting induced by the surgery. The understanding of this fact has taken us back to the place of fasting as a treatment for diabetes before the discovery of insulin.

There are significant side effects of weight-loss surgery. Doctors prefer to use this surgery only on extremely obese patients. Some may weigh 500 or 600 pounds. Weight-loss surgery can save their lives in many cases. Weight-loss surgery is not recommended as treatment for diabetes, but the fact remains that the surgery can reverse type 2 diabetes.

Stomach bypass patients are put on a special low-calorie, low-carb diet before and after surgery. The overall long-term success of their weight loss depends on how they modify their eating behavior after their weight-loss surgery.

Fasting

*If you are going on a fast, you should consult your medical
care professional before attempting this strategy to lose
weight or reverse your diabetes. This is really important if
you are being treated with prescribed medications or
insulin to lower your blood sugar levels.*

Different approaches to fasting without surgery have also proven to
reverse diabetes. A complete food fast is where no solid food is eaten at all.
A juice fast is where no solid food is eaten, but juices are allowed. Juice
fasts are not recommended for someone with diabetes. Fasts can last for a
few hours or a few days. Many people are required to fast 12 to 14 hours
before taking laboratory tests.

The human body can go without food for about 40 days, but it cannot
survive without water for more than two or three days. If you choose to
fast, you should drink plenty of water. Fasting without drinking water is
not recommended. You should drink plenty of water while fasting.

Fasting will affect your blood sugar levels. You should always continue to
monitor your blood sugar levels while fasting to avoid dangerously low
blood sugar levels. If you are on medications like insulin, you should never
risk your personal safety while fasting. Your doctor can tell you how to
decrease your diabetes medications or insulin during your fast.

If you are going to do a total food fast, you should begin some type of
transition diet before you just stop eating for a few days. Some transition
diets begin by eliminating meat and dairy products and eating only fresh
fruit and vegetables for a week or 10 days before the fast begins.

Many individuals routinely fast for 7 or 10 days and find it beneficial to
clear their minds and improve their health. After three or four days of a
complete food fast, most people see their blood sugar levels stabilize at a
constant level. Because no solid food or carbohydrates are being eaten, the
body shifts to burning ketones from fat and other tissues instead of

glucose. Usually, hunger craving will cease after two or three days on a complete food fast.

Fasting is often useful as a strategy for detoxification. Fasting induces the body to detoxify itself. Toxins stored in fat cells are released from fat cells, that are being used for energy. Drinking plenty of water helps to flush these toxins from your body.

People who are unused to fasting will often experience, headaches, dizziness and weakness as a result of detoxification. This is sometimes accompanied by flu-like symptoms. This is from the body restoring itself from years of unhealthy eating. This effect may last a day or longer.

Dr. Mercola has a great understanding of the medical benefits of fasting. Additional information about how fasting can help reverse or prevent type 2 diabetes can be found on the Internet using this link: http://articles.mercola.com/sites/articles/archive/2016/10/16/complete-guide-fasting.aspx

Intermittent Fasting

Intermittent Fasting and Longevity

Intermittent fasting has proven to be an effective short-term strategy to lose weight and reverse many instances of type 2 diabetes. Restricting or reducing the calories you eat over the long-term may also be an effective strategy to increase the length of your life by many years.

Studies at Cornell University on rats in the 1930s demonstrated that a 30 to 40 percent reduction in calorie intake could extend their lifespan by a third or more. Rats that ate less lived longer and were less likely to develop cancer and other diseases as they aged.

Intermittent fasting has periods of fasting and periods of eating. It does not involve restrictions on food, but only on the time the food is eaten. The most popular form of intermittent fasting is not eating breakfast. This will go on for a predetermined time. The trick here is not to double up on your eating during the other regular meal times.

In 1945 University of Chicago scientists demonstrated that feeding rats every other day extended the life span of the rats as much as did the caloric restriction of every meal by 30 to 40 percent. These scientists reported that intermittent fasting delayed the development of diseases that cause death. Animals given less food have fewer tumors and other age-related problems.

Studies on rice, mice, rhesus monkeys and other animals have provided life-extending results. Studies to determine caloric restriction on humans would take 100 years because humans have a much longer lifespan than most lab animals. One can assume that the results for increasing the lifespans of lab animals would also pertain to humans.

Intermittent fasting and total fasting can help you extend your life by many years. You could also experience a better quality of life and less age-related diseases and age-related complications.

Reported Benefits of Intermittent Fasting

Here are some of the results from intermittent fasting studies performed on humans:

- Reduced fasting glucose (blood sugar) levels
- Reduced after meal (post-prandial) glucose (blood sugar) levels
- Increased insulin sensitivity
- Increased fat burning and weight loss
- Reduced bad cholesterol
- Increased good cholesterol
- Reduced triglycerides
- Reduced blood pressure
- Reduced inflammation

Intermittent Fasting as a Long-Term Strategy

Intermittent fasting can be an effective long-term strategy to maintain your weight and live a healthier lifestyle after you complete short-term diabetes reversal programs or other weight loss programs.

Specialized diabetes reversal programs like the Newcastle diet and related Diabetes Destroyer Program can be used to jumpstart your weight loss and reverse type 2 diabetes. These strategies can be completed in a few weeks.

After successful completion of one of these short-term programs, you might consider using an intermittent fasting strategy as a long-term strategy to maintain your health and extend your lifespan. This would insure you did not lose the benefits of the short-term plans you used to manage or reverse your diabetes and provide many of the other proven benefits of intermittent fasting.

Here is a useful link to Dr. Julian Whitaker's Website with some information about reversing type 2 diabetes with intermittent fasting. He calls his intermittent fasting program a Mini-Fast Program.

http://www.drwhitaker.com/reverse-diabetes-with-the-mini-fast-program/

Magic Pills, Magic Exercises and False Promises

Some diabetes reversal strategies make outrageous claims. Some promise that diabetes is 100% reversible when it is not. Those who make 100% reversible promises about diabetes are making unrealistic claims that play on the emotions and create false hopes. No one should claim that type 2 diabetes is 100% reversible.

Type 2 diabetes may be 80%-90% reversible with diet and exercise changes during its early stages. However, it is more unlikely to be reversed if someone has had it for 10 years or longer.   For those situations where complete diabetes reversal does not take place, reversal programs may still be useful to lower blood sugar levels. This may result in the reduction of the amount of insulin and other medications being used. In these situations, diabetes symptoms may have been lessened, but they have not been reversed.

Some weight loss strategies make claims that some magic pills can be taken to cause you to lose weight and belly fat almost effortlessly within a couple of days. They may even warn you not to take too much to keep you from losing weight too fast. These claims are false and misleading.

This book has already discussed how weight is gained or lost. True weight loss from losing body fat depends on eating fewer calories than the number calories you burn up with physical activity and bodily functions. There are no magic pills that will burn up fat in a short amount of time.

You cannot target one particular kind of fat over another. You cannot specify belly fat or arm fat. People with different body shapes will each lose fat differently. Eat less and move more, and you will lose fat. Keep losing fat until your problem area disappears.

No exercise will burn up pure fat. It takes many hours of exercise over a period of days to actually burn fat. A trained athlete may burn up to 700 calories or more an hour while exercising. If it were even possible, at this rate it would take this athlete almost 5 hours to burn up a pound of fat. This is not realistic because exercise first uses the existing energy stored in the muscles and liver before it starts to convert fat into energy.

There are no magic exercises that will cause you to cure diabetes in only a few seconds a day. If you stopped eating altogether during your exercising and burned 2,000 calories a day, it would take three and one-half days to burn the 7,000 calories in two pounds of fat. However, 30 minutes to 60 minutes of daily exercise will do wonders to help you control your blood sugar and lose weight. It may take several weeks, but you will start seeing results from exercising more and eating less.

Exercise does change your ability to burn energy more efficiently. Consistent exercise will increase your metabolism, lower your insulin resistance and control your blood sugar. It will also help you lose weight.

Unfortunately, there are no magic pills or magic exercises to reverse type 2 diabetes overnight. However, consistent exercise habits, when combined with a low-carb, very low-calorie, low-carb diet, can reverse most type 2 diabetes in as little as eight weeks.

Don't Throw the Baby Out with the Bath Water

Some diabetes reversal programs make unrealistic claims in their marketing presentations, but these programs can actually contain some valuable information. In these cases, you should not throw out the baby with the bath water. In other words, you should disregard some of the marketing hype and look at the program's action steps. If you look under the hood (bonnet), you will actually find the program's plans and actions steps are quite useful. This makes the programs worth keeping.

Losing weight, improving your physical conditioning and gaining better control of your blood sugar levels will take effort and time. It cannot happen overnight. However, in just a few weeks you can start seeing real progress towards achieving your goals.

There are many documented testimonies of success from the Diabetes Destroyer and Diabetes60 Systems. They are real success stories from real people who have followed their programs step-by-step. That is why I recommend them. I have included links to these program in the Additional Resources section at the end of this book.

These diabetes reversal programs have been very successful with people who follow them step-by-step. They will produce results, but only if you put in the time and effort to follow them.

The Diabetes Destroyer and Diabetes60 System can help you lose weight, get in shape, control your blood sugar and may help you to completely reverse type 2 diabetes. Many times significant results can be seen in several weeks.

However, in some cases, these programs may not reverse type 2 diabetes completely. This may be particularly true for those who have had the disease longer than 10 years. These programs will not completely reverse diabetes when the pancreas is unable to produce sufficient insulin. These programs will also not reverse type 2 diabetes for anyone who does not put forth much time and effort into following the plans.

Final Words–Take Action and Don't Give Up!

Stick with it!

New Year's resolutions are seldom kept. After the first of the year, many people will start going to the gym and the parking lot out front is full. Many people have made a resolution to get in shape and lose weight. Then, after three or four weeks, you will notice that the gym is not as full, and the parking lot has plenty of empty parking spaces.

Human nature is what it is. Most people will quickly give up trying to keep their New Year's resolutions. Their effort to follow through on their resolution quickly fades out. Good intentions give way to failure. There was no commitment, no dedication and no discipline to the complete the resolution.

Commitment means you ae willing to spend your time an effort towards accomplishing your goals. Commitment means you dedicate yourself to an activity until it is finished. There is a no difference between wishful thinking, good intentions and SMART goals if no commitment is made and no actions are taken to reach your goal.

SMART goals, developing strategies and following action steps are more powerful than resolutions because they are **S**pecific, **M**easurable, **A**ccountable, **R**ealistic, and **T**imely. However, SMART goals and action plans can break down and only be good intentions, or wishful thinking, if you do make the commitment, and make the effort, to complete the action steps.

Take Action with the Keys
You Have Been Given

Suppose you have been given the keys to a new car. You are excited about your new car. You want everyone to know about what you have been given. Let us suppose further that you go out into the parking lot and jump on the hood of your new car and shout as loud as you can, "These are the keys to my new car. These keys will start my new car. I have been given the keys to this new car!"

Just shouting about the keys to a new car means nothing unless you get in the car and use the keys. It is not good enough to have good intentions and tell the world you have the keys unless you use them to get in the car and drive the car wherever you want to go.

You need to take action with the keys you have in your hand, or you will just look silly shouting about it. Your commitment to use the keys and to take action is what makes the difference is getting the benefit and enjoyment from driving your new car.

It takes time to accomplish goals. If you go in the gym and do not have a definite date to accomplish your goal, or if you do not have some sort of measurement to determine how far you have gone, you have no Specific, Measurable, Accountable, Realistic and Timely goal.

Once you set your goals, strategies and action steps, stay with the plan until your reach your goals. If you did not develop a good plan at first, revise it so that you can stick with it.

This is where accountability comes into play. If you are falling off your plan, it is good to have someone else other than yourself to hold you accountable to reach your goals. Measuring your progress, and being held accountable, will go a long way in helping you keep your commitment to achieving your goals.

If You Fall Down–Get Right Back Up!

Children fall when they are first learning to walk. A baby's first steps are preceded by falls. Children who learn to ice skate, ski or ride a bicycle experience failure at first, but they keep on trying until they succeed. Cut yourself some slack. If you fail to lose weight or control your blood sugar, get up and try again until you succeed.

Often those that succeed are not the most gifted or the most talented. They are not the best planners, but they are determined to never quit. Once you quit you are defeated. Keep going, and if you fail, get up and try again.

Many times it is not the plan that failed–it is the commitment to follow the plan that failed. Do not quit before you accomplish your goals. If you fall down, pick yourself up and try again. Keep following your plan and working towards your goals. Then, you will achieve the success you desire.

Sedentary lifestyles and unhealthy eating habits are not conditions that just happened suddenly. They involve habits that have taken years to form. Reversing diabetes is not something that you can do overnight. However, making a commitment to take action and follow a good plan will go a long way to getting you some very good results, and in some cases, this will happen in just a few weeks.

Short-term goal achievements along with long-term lifestyle changes are worth the commitment and effort. Living a healthier lifestyle will improve your quality of life, and you will be around longer for those you love and those who love you.

Take Responsibility for Your Health

You are responsible for the amount and type of food you choose to eat. You are also responsible for sitting on the couch or moving your body to burn up calories. You do not have to eat unhealthy foods. You can make the right choices when it comes to putting the right food in your mouth and exercising more often.

Doctors' advice and drugs can help control blood sugar levels and prolong your life. They can help most people deal with the effects of bad eating habits and lack of exercise. Doctors can help treat and control the symptoms of diabetes with drugs and medicines. However, your goal should go beyond controlling the symptoms of diabetes with medications. Your goal should be to make healthy lifestyle decisions and reduce or eliminate the need for drugs and medications through diet and exercise.

Your personal commitment to make the necessary changes to live a healthier lifestyle is a powerful force that leads to change. Exercising more and eating less will help you control your blood sugar levels, lose weight, and lower your insulin resistance.

Exercising more and eating fewer carbs will deal with the underlying problems that contribute to most instances of prediabetes and type 2 diabetes. Dealing with those things that contribute to diabetes is better than only treating the symptoms.

Results will vary for each person depending upon how dedicated they are to changing their lifestyles. It is up to each person, not their doctor, to take responsibility for their own actions. It is up to each person, not their doctor, to make a commitment to follow an action plan that includes more exercise and eating fewer carbs.

If you keep working towards your goals, you will achieve success. If you do not have any goals, and if you do not work towards your goals, things will not change. If you do not take responsibility for your health, things will only get worse as time goes by.

Take Action Now!

Modern science has given us the knowledge that prediabetes can be prevented from turning into type 2 diabetes, and most type 2 diabetes symptoms can be reversed with diet and exercise changes.

Knowledge is power. Take this knowledge and apply it to your situation or to the situation of someone you care for. If enough people take action one person at a time, life will be made better for millions of people with type 2 diabetes and millions more with prediabetes.

This book was written to help you understand what diabetes is, how prediabetes and type 2 diabetes can be reversed, and why you should never ignore it. Diabetes is not a death sentence. You do have positive options to choose from.

If you have prediabetes or type 2 diabetes, there is hope for you and a plan for you to control your blood sugar levels through diet and exercise. It is possible that you will be one of the millions of people who can reverse prediabetes or type 2 diabetes and not have to take diabetes medicines or insulin.

A good place to start is by selecting one of the action plans at the end of this book. Then, invest the time and effort to follow the action plans. You can achieve great results and accomplish your goals like many others who have set good examples for you to follow.

Make a quality decision right now to take responsibility for your health. Then, immediately follow this decision with corresponding actions that lead to a healthier life.

The choice to live a healthier life is yours to make! You can make your choice right now and begin to take immediate action!

****

Author's Note: This is the first edition of this book. If you see any errors or typos, please let me know. I would appreciate any help in making it better for future readers of the next revision.

Thanks for reading this book. I welcome your feedback and testimonies about how this information has helped you.

James Strand

April 2017

You can contact me, the author, at this email address:

james1@reversediabetes101.com

****

****

**A Kindle version of this book
is also available on amazon.com**

****

Additional Resources

Two of the Best Type 2 Diabetes Action Plans

Diabetes Destroyer–Step-by-Step
Type 2 Diabetes Reversal Diet Plan

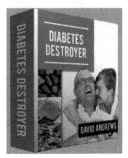

http://reversediabetes101.com/1

Diabetes Destroyer developed by David Andrews, a former diabetic and chef, is a complete package for reversing most cases of type 2 diabetes. The focus is on an 8-week diet plan that provides excellent nutrition and delicious recipes.'

The sales presentation is a little long-winded and skimpy on action steps, but the product will work. After purchase, you will find a lot of good information and detailed action steps. This should be the first action plan you implement.

When this action plan is strictly followed, it provides better blood sugar control and reverses a large percentage of type 2 diabetes cases.

The 8-week Diabetes Destroyer when combined with the 8-week Diabetes 60 System provides a powerful two-fold strategy to control blood sugar and reduce insulin resistance.

Diabetes 60 System–Step-by-Step
Type 2 Diabetes Exercise Plan

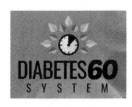

http://reversediabetes101.com/2

Developed by Dr. Ryan Shelton to help manage diabetes, the Diabetes 60 System has several aspects, but the exercises are the strongest part of the package. The exercises will take at least 60 seconds each. The program will require a few minutes a day. It is not a 60-second program.

Diabetes Destroyer Program and Diabetes 60 System Action Plan Discounts and Bonuses

Discounts

For readers of this edition of the book, I have a special discount order page for the Diabetes Destroyer program and the Diabetes 60 System. I will send you a link to this and you will save $10 on each one of these packages.

To get the discounts by email send your request to:

discounts@diabetes101.com

Bonuses

I have created two detailed action plans to show you how to quickly implement the Diabetes Destroyer program and the Diabetes 60 System. The Diabetes Destroyer program and the Diabetes 60 System include a lot of material. My action plans will walk you through the most important things to do first. This will help you achieve the results you are looking for faster.

If you email me a copy of your purchase receipt for the Diabetes Destroyer and or the purchase receipt for the Diabetes 60 System, I will email you the action plan for each receipt you send. You must use one of the links provided in this book to purchase the products for this offer to be valid.

– James

Email address: **bonuses@diabetes101.com**

60-Day Money-Back Guarantee

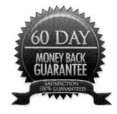

All our product vendors provide a 60-Day-Money-Back-Guarantee. They will guarantee your satisfaction with the product, or they will refund your money.

More Diabetes-Related Action Plans

Eat Stop Eat–Simple Intermittent Fasting Diet

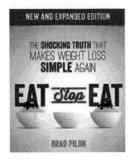

http://reversediabetes101.com/3

Here's what this program will do for you: increase your fat-burning hormone, control your hunger hormone, help you lose weight, decrease your stress hormone and increase your brain function and concentration. There are no complicated rules to follow.

The Keto Beginning–Fat-Burning Meals, Shopping Lists and Recipes

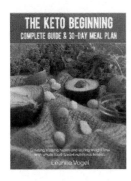

http://reversediabetes101.com/4

30-day meal plans with daily recipes that are ready in 15 minutes or less. Weekly shopping lists. Whole foods based low-carbohydrate approach to nutritional ketosis that burns body fat instead of glucose.

Metabolic Cooking–Quick Easy Fat-burning Recipes

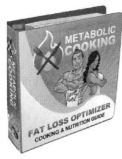

http://reversediabetes101.com/5

Professional fitness coach, nutritionist and competitive bodybuilder, David Ruel, shows you the simplest and fastest way to prepare delicious fat-burning meals. Enough recipes are included so you can eat healthy food every day for the rest of your life. There are 250 fat torching recipes included to enhance your diet and burn fat.

7 Steps to Health–Scientists Reveal the Truth about Diabetes

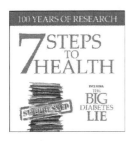

http://reversediabetes101.com/6

Excellent background and scientific based evidence about type 2 diabetes. The writers may go a little overboard on the conspiracy angle, but the diabetes reversal 30-day plan is solid and provides good information on nutrition for diabetes.

Neuropathy Solution Program

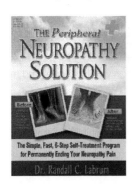

http://reversediabetes101.com/7

This simple 6-step program from Dr. Randall Labrum shows you how to end chronic peripheral neuropathy and diabetic nerve pain without drugs, surgery or guesswork.

Never Grow Old Functional Fitness Solution

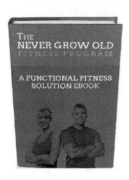

http://reversediabetes101.com/8

Feel 20 years younger in 20 minutes a day, three times a week. Eliminate the pain and agony of getting older while improving your ability to do what you love with this easy at home system that makes you feel 20 years younger. This fitness program was created by Ph.D. experts on aging.

Smartphone Diabetes Apps

FREE TRIAL

Noom Weight-Loss Coaching Program and Smartphone App

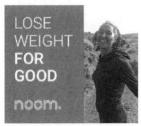

http://reversediabetes101.com/9

This is a weight-loss program with coaching. The free smartphone app, Noom Coach, includes calorie counting and weight tracking. Fill out the brief survey and receive a customized plan for healthy weight loss. The free coaching is available after the brief survey. They also have a free step-tracking app, Noom Walk Pedometer. Noom, Inc. has 45 million users worldwide.

iHealth Smart Glucose Meter
A Great Accountability Tool

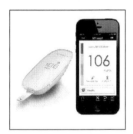

http://reversediabetes101.com/10

Wirelessly connects to your smartphone by Bluetooth. Includes USB charging cable, lance, lancets and case. The free iHealth App is available from the Google Play Store or iTunes. You can track and share your results with your doctor and others. This is a great accountability tool. $29.99 + Shipping.

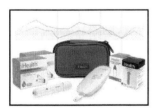

If you buy the iHealth Smart Gluco-Monitor Bundle, you will save 15%. You will get the meter package plus 1 box of lancets (50 count), 1 control solution, and 2 boxes of test strips (100 count) $56.99+Free Shipping (US).

To see this offer scroll down to the bottom of the page
http://reversediabetes101.com/10

Diabetes Tests and Other Lab Tests

Walk-In-Lab–US Local Labs

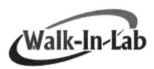

http://reversediabetes101.com/11

Order a test online. Visit a local lab. Get your results online in a couple of days. No doctor's orders are necessary. The tests are confidential and competitively priced. The link above brings up the tests specifically related to diabetes: A1c, plasma (serum) glucose test, two-hour glucose tolerance test, urine test.

Other tests that are useful for diabetes are available: cholesterol, triglycerides, CMP (comprehensive metabolic panel). There are also hundreds of other confidential medical lab tests you can order for yourself.

Diet and Weight Loss Action Plans

3 Week Diet–Melt Away Several Pounds in Just 21 Days

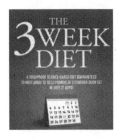

http://reversediabetes101.com/12

The 3 Week Diet is a foolproof, science-based diet that is guaranteed to melt away several pounds of body fat in 21 days. Discover the list of unique foods that help you burn fat fast.

Fat-Burning Kitchen and 23 Day Fat-Burning Blueprint

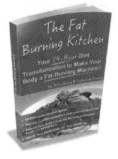

http: //reversediabetes101.com/13

Discover exactly what bread, milk, sugar and vegetable oils do to your body, and why it is not your fault if you cannot lose weight. This blueprint will decrease your risks for diabetes, Alzheimer's and cancer.

Coconut Oil Secret Tropical Superfood and Beauty Bundle

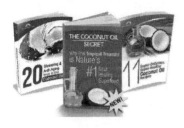

http://reversediabetes101.com/14

Researchers have discovered when unrefined coconut oil is part of an everyday diet, there is less obesity and fewer lifestyle diseases like diabetes and cancer. You will learn the nine reasons to use coconut oil daily–three of these are shocking. Plus, four common yet dangerous oils you should never eat if you want to heal, beautify and restore your body.

Unusual Red Smoothie–Four Red Ingredients–Detox–and Eat Less

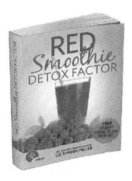

http://reversediabetes101.com/15

Doctor of Naturopathy and weight-loss expert, Liz Swann Miller, has developed a delicious method called the Red Smoothie Detox Factor. She will show you how to swiftly liberate your body from the toxins in your body from eating processed foods. She also shows you how it is better to eat real food, and you will eat less without feeling deprived.

21-Day Sugar Detox Program

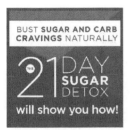

http://reversediabetes101.com/16

The 21-Day Sugar Detox is a comprehensive, simple and effective program to break the chains of sugar and carb cravings. The Premium program package includes two printed books with easy to make recipes. You will also receive a membership to their website with the Quick Start Guide and more information. There are also a few free resources there, too.

Old School New Body–Look Years Younger for Men and Women

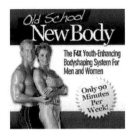

http://reversediabetes101.com/17

Old School New Body gives you five steps to look 10 years younger. This breakthrough program shows you how to slow the aging process, sculpt your body to look like you want it to look–and do it in just 90 minutes a week.

Paleo Recipe Books–Regain Your Health, Energy, Vitality and Power

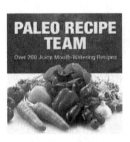

http://reversediabetes101.com/18

These paleo recipes are designed around the concept that simpler is better. A long time ago, humans ate food that was simple and unprocessed. The paleo diet is starch-free, grain-free, dairy-free, refined sugar-free and free of additives you cannot pronounce. The recipe books include recipes for snacks, omelets, meats, soups, salads and desserts. A few additional paleo guidebooks are included as a bonus. The recipes are easy to make, highly nutritional and delicious.

High Blood Pressure Exercise Program

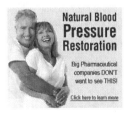

http://reversediabetes101.com/19

This unique hypertension program by Blue Heron Health News can lower your blood pressure to 120/80 or less with simple exercises that take 9 minutes a day

Diabetes Questions and Answers
by Shawn Bao, M.D.

> ## Diabetes Questions
> ## and Answers
>
> Shunzhong Shawn Bao, M.D.
>
> Endocrinology and
> Diabetes Specialist

If you have diabetes, or if you have a family member with diabetes, this is why you need to read Dr. Shawn Bao's new book *Diabetes Questions and Answers.*

For most people, a trip to a doctor's office means spending time in a crowded waiting room. Many people also spend time traveling from out of town to visit their doctor. People spend a lot of time going to see their doctors, and when you are finally able to see your doctor, he or she only spends a few minutes with you.

What if it were somehow possible for you to spend hours with an expert doctor who has worked with diabetes patients for many years? What would it be like if you could pick his brain to find all the nuggets of wisdom he has learned over many years of treating patients with diabetes? What questions would you ask him?

This is now possible with the new book *Diabetes Questions and Answers* by Dr. Shawn Bao. He is an Endocrinologist and an expert in providing medical care for people with diabetes. His new book contains 400 of the most commonly asked questions about diabetes.

This book provides you with a treasure trove of information about the practical day-to-day solutions for patients living with and managing diabetes. It condenses questions from hundreds of patients and hundreds of answers into one useful book.

With this book, it is as if you are looking over his shoulder as he meets with patients and answers their questions. You may be able to find this information during 400 visits with your doctor, but you will not have to make 400 appointments. You can save your time and order this book now with all the valuable information it provides.

Here are some of the questions Dr. Bao has answered:

- What 10 things do I need to know after being newly diagnosed with diabetes?
- What 10 questions should I ask my insurance company about diabetes treatment options?
- What10 things should I discuss with my family about diabetes?
- What should I eat, and when do I eat if I have diabetes?
- What do I need to know about diabetes and exercise?
- What should I do if I have high or low blood sugar?
- What are the different treatments for type 1 and type 2 diabetes?
- What are the different kinds of diabetes medicines and insulins?
- What do I need to know about glucose meters and strips?
- What are the different tests for diabetes?
- What do I need to know about diabetes foot care and foot problems?
- How do I live with somebody who has diabetes?
- Can diabetes cause sexual dysfunction? If so, what can I do about it?
- I am planning to travel. What tips do you have?
- The holidays are coming up. Do you have any tips for holiday eating?

You will find all the answers to these questions and more in Dr. Shawn Bao's book *Diabetes Questions and Answers*. For more information email:

drbaobook@reversediabetes101.com

Made in United States
Troutdale, OR
07/29/2023

11661265R00066